The
Repetitive
Strain Injury
Sourcebook

by
Sandra Peddie
with
Craig H. Rosenberg, M.D.

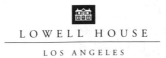

LOWELL HOUSE

LOS ANGELES

CONTEMPORARY BOOKS

CHICAGO

Library of Congress Cataloging-in Publication-Data
Peddie, Sandra.
    The repetitive strain injury sourcebook / by Sandra Peddie,
with Craig H. Rosenberg.
        p.   cm.
    Includes biographical references and index.
    ISBN 1-56565-791-8
    II. Title.
    RD97.6.P435   1997
    617.1—dc21
                                                            97-34717
                                                                CIP

Requests for such permissions should be addressed to:

        Lowell House
        2020 Avenue of the Stars, Suite 300
        Los Angeles, CA 90067

Lowell House books can be purchased at special discounts when
ordered in bulk for premiums and special sales.

Publisher: Jack Artenstein
Associate Publisher, Lowell House Adult: Bud Sperry
Director of Publishing Services: Rena Copperman
Managing Editor: Maria Magallanes
Text design: Robert S. Tinnon

Manufactured in the United States of America
10 9 8 7 6 5 4 3 2 1

CONTENTS

�֍

ACKNOWLEDGMENTS

I would like to thank the following people for their time and assistance: Ginger Rothe, Jackie Ross, Dr. David Thompson of Portola Associates, Susan Nobel of Mt. Sinai Medical Center, Stephanie Barnes of the Association for Repetitive Motion Syndromes, Dr. John H. Hung of Health Psychology Consultants, Richard Brandenstein and Victor Fusco of Scheine, Fusco, Brandenstein and Rada, Michael Gauf of CTD News, Chris Leick of Health Care Keyboards, Hilary Marcus of the Massachusetts Coalition on New Office Technology, David LeGrande of the Communication Workers of America, Nancy Lessin of the Massachusetts Coalition for Occupation Health and Safety, the Human Factors and Ergonomics Society, the 9 to 5 National Association of Working Women, the National Institute of Occupational Safety and Health and all the people with RSI who graciously agreed to share their experiences with me for this book. I would also like to thank my husband for his support and his typing.

FOREWORD

RSI can be a source of fear and anxiety to someone who performs repetitive tasks on a routine basis. There has been an extraordinary amount of sensationalism associated with it. I feel a responsibility not only to my patients but to others to strip away the myths and provide the groundwork for educating people about RSI.

Listening to war stories from a buddy in the washroom can be dangerous. As a result of the growing prevalence of RSI, there are many self-proclaimed experts in the field. The purpose of this book is to provide the reader with a better understanding about the facts and issues related to RSI. I also have a warning for the reader: Do not use this book for the purpose of making a self-diagnosis.

I have been treating patients with RSI for more than ten years. Through the years, my knowledge and appreciation of RSI and its risk factors continue to evolve. Since then, I have gained a much better understanding of RSI and its associated risk factors. Early on, it was easy to blame only workplace factors. Over time, I have come to understand the importance of taking a global look at a patient's situation. Many factors are associated with RSI, and those in the workplace are only part of a broader picture. I have come to appreciate the importance of other factors, such as avocational activities.

Identifying causative factors is not an easy process. It takes time and effort. In some situations, I have asked patients to keep a diary of activities, no matter how mundane, that they are performing. This exercise is extremely helpful in cases when I am unable to ascertain a cause-and-effect relationship from the information provided during an interview with a new patient. I am continually amazed at the naiveté of people regarding activities they perform regularly without being aware of their repetitive nature.

We all complain about time constraints. Physicians are no different. Some remarkable technological advancements have also been made in the area of diagnostic testing. A high-tech approach should never be substituted for taking a history and physical examination. The patient's history is the most important information that a doctor can obtain in order to guide him toward making an accurate diagnosis and establishing an appropriate treatment plan. A properly taken history is also the first step in establishing physician-patient rapport, and it should encourage open communication. Forms may be helpful, but the physician must verbally review and clarify the information verbally with the patient. There are no compromises.

There is a time and a place for high-tech diagnostic testing. However, there is no substitute for clinical knowledge and experience. The shotgun approach of ordering extensive testing early on is not recommended. Many tests are highly sensitive and have a low specificity. This means that there is a risk of making a falsely positive diagnosis. Falsely positive findings can potentially raise the patient's anxiety level, and lead to unnecessary therapeutic intervention. Diagnostic testing does have a place and should be utilized under the right circumstances.

I believe in a holistic approach. My chosen field of specialization, physical medicine and rehabilitation, is unique in this regard. Physiatrists are taught to gain a comprehensive understanding of their patients. We treat people, not diseases. We learn to evaluate a patient's impairment, disability, and function.

I've often been surprised by how much doctors can learn

from their patients. Once, I had a patient who had a case of carpal tunnel syndrome that was serious enough to consider surgery. Unwilling to undergo surgery, the patient opted to pursue conservative (nonsurgical) treatment, which was against my better judgment. The carpal tunnel syndrome cleared up. This is not an uncommon occurrence in medicine. Many of our current standards of practice are based upon positive outcomes of patients who didn't follow our recommendations.

However, physicians have a responsibility to be able to statistically reproduce a treatment intervention before making recommendations to other patients. Treatment should not be based upon anecdotal findings. We must remain open-minded and use every opportunity to learn from all situations. I have learned that the decision tree I utilize to guide my course of treatment recommendations can grow extra branches.

As doctors, we must try to understand the nature of the person we are treating. There are some people you can give advice to, and they'll take it with a grain of salt and never follow up. I try to sense when that will happen. There are others who hang on my every word of advice, and I have become concerned that they may be overreading the situation. Some patients can also be angry and tell me (directly or indirectly), I will not take responsibility for my condition; it is my employer's problem. But this is not a situation where the patient and/or worker can simply go along for the ride. You don't get better unless you want to get better. Patients are important members of the treatment team. Do not allow emotion to cloud your judgment and good sense. It helps to put things into perspective and focus on the bigger picture. Take an active role on the treatment team and help it set realistic and measurable short- and long-term goals that will address work- and nonwork-related problems.

For the most part, people want to be productive in all aspects of their lives. There is so much physical and emotional stress to just keep your life on track, the more understanding you have, the better. Different diagnoses require different treatments. RSI is complex and sometimes psychological intervention may be needed. It's not taboo.

People who have been diagnosed with RSI often experience many emotions, much like the stages Elisabeth Kübler-Ross describes as part of the mourning process—denial, bargaining, anger, depression, and resignation. While grieving is natural, it is important to work through the phases in order to start down the road of healing. It is important for physicians to have an understanding of the grieving process in order to help patients work their way through it. While progressing through the stages of grief, psychosomatic symptoms such as body aches, emotional tension, poor sleep, and fatigue are not uncommon. Eventually, an emotional balance will occur.

Compassion is an important quality, but it should not cloud a physician's advice and judgment. It's hard to create a wall between the physician and the patient. A relationship develops, and the doctor must accept the role as the patient's advocate. We take the Hippocratic Oath. We are ethically bound to do the right thing. The physician as a leader, based upon his specialized knowledge and experience, has a responsibility to his patients to guide them in a forthright manner and to make recommendations based upon scientific principles and established standards of best practice. Trying to create a fine balance can be difficult at times, especially if doctors must tell their patient something that they may not want to hear. A relationship built upon open communication and trust is so important.

Patients do touch our lives. I've been touched by patients who refused to be overcome by their condition, patients who were courageous and fought back with undaunting tenacity. These people are my real-life heroes. They have accepted the challenge to move forward with their lives, which is much harder than it sounds.

As a physiatrist, I have come to appreciate that life cannot be neatly planned. You cannot bring back what once was. It takes time to heal a painful wound. Address each situation as it arises, and make the best of it. It takes courage to make major life and career changes. It takes strength and determination to move on with your life after you have been stricken with a disability. It's a special moment when I see patients who have put forth their best effort and successfully completed treatment. I derive hope and joy from assisting them achieve their successes. This is a measure of my success as a doctor.

I have also learned to respect the fortitude of the human spirit. As a family-oriented person, I understand the importance of raising children. For some of my patients this idea did not seem prudent. This was a dilemma because I couldn't advise them not to fulfill their dream. It was a difficult process, and it required devotion on their part to make it work. Attention and ingenuity were needed to develop alternative methods for addressing parental obligations. In the end, watching these children flourish and seeing the look of contentment on their parents' faces has been a touching and rewarding experience.

Undoubtedly, prevention is the best treatment. Realizing that RSI is cumulative in nature, a proactive approach to study and change the way we treat patients is essential. Patients must be open-minded and understand that in addition to identifying and correcting work-related factors, nonwork-related factors must be addressed if they want to get better or avoid becoming disabled. The concept is to identify all causative factors and to be committed to changing the way we treat patients in order to minimize the physical and emotional stresses that can either cause or complicate RSI.

A book like this is long overdue. Again, use it to gain a better understanding of RSI.

CRAIG H. ROSENBERG, M.D.

PREFACE

❧

Although no one claims to have all the answers on Repetitive Strain Injury, information is available to help you prevent it and take care of it. This book will take you through that information, chapter by chapter.

A broad overview of RSI, from its history to today's political fight over ergonomic regulations, is discussed in chapter 1, along with its human cost, as related through individual stories.

Chapter 2 explains the various medical disorders that fall into the category of RSI. One of the most common is carpal tunnel syndrome, a compression of the nerve that runs through the wrist into the hand. Many people use the term interchangeably with Repetitive Strain Injury, but it is, in fact, only one manifestation of it. Others include nerve disorders, tendinitis, tenosynovitis, ganglion cysts, tennis elbow, thoracic outlet syndrome, Raynaud's disease, fibromyalgia, and writer's cramp.

Chapters 3 and 4 look at the causes of RSI and who is at risk. This is a controversial topic, as people jockey for position in lawsuits and fights over regulation, but researchers have linked it to a number of factors, including posture, repetition, force, workstation and equipment design, job design, vibration, and stress. There may be individual risk factors at work as well, such as genetic predispositions and hobbies. Understanding the cause and risk factors is one way to prevent the problem without blaming the victim.

Prevention is the focus of chapter 5, which offers detailed information on how to prevent RSI from happening to you—from making physical changes in your workstation to changing the way you work. Some people with early symptoms of RSI have made the kinds of ergonomic changes discussed here and have seen their symptoms disappear. Others with more serious injuries have been able to guard themselves against relapse by making such changes. This chapter focuses on computer workstations because of the widespread use of computers at work and at home.

Chapters 6, 7, and 8 discuss finding the right doctor and available treatment options. Recovery can be a long road if you are seriously injured. It is important to find a knowledgeable doctor with whom you feel comfortable. Just as important is getting treatment as soon as possible. The longer you put it off, the worse the condition gets.

Chapter 9 looks at some of the alternative therapies tried by people with RSI. This exploration is not meant as an endorsement of any particular therapy; it is only a brief description of some therapies people say have helped them. As with any treatment option, if you decide to try one, discuss it with your doctor.

Coping with the injury, both physically and emotionally, is covered in chapters 10 and 11. Few people, unless they've experienced the injury themselves, understand the sheer physical difficulty in doing simple tasks or the emotional roller coaster that people with RSI experience. Little information is available on these topics, yet there is a desperate need for it.

The financial and legal implications of RSI are discussed in chapters 12 and 13. Because this injury threatens the ability to work, financial worries are a big problem for many sufferers. Chapter 12 explains worker's compensation, disability, and other benefits. Chapter 13 details how to protect your rights, which can be trampled by the system.

Chapter 14 talks about change: how RSI can change your life in positive ways, as well as the broader political changes that are occurring.

The epilogue includes personal accounts from the author and her husband on how RSI affected their lives. It is followed by a glossary and appendix, with detailed information on where you can get more information.

The information in this book is intended to help you make informed decisions. It is not meant to substitute for the advice of medical professionals. No medication, treatment, or exercise done for RSI should be undertaken without first consulting a qualified medical professional.

CHAPTER 1

RSI: COMING TO A HOME NEAR YOU

❈

You may have it and not even know it.

Symptoms of Repetitive Strain Injury (RSI), the fastest-growing workplace injury in the country, are insidious. They often sneak up on you, catching you unaware. You'll probably feel them hours after you've finished the activity that actually caused them. Sometimes they flare up in an instant, without warning. Other times they explode only after months of occasional twinges and aches that you've likely dismissed as no big deal. Or maybe you were simply too busy to think about them.

The symptoms run the gamut, from a little numbness and tingling in the hands and fingertips to an aching in the neck and shoulders to outright burning pain in your forearms. They can be a mere annoyance or become a crippling injury. Because they mimic the symptoms of so many other conditions, from Lyme disease to the simple aches and pains of growing older, it's easy to confuse them with something else. But make no mistake, RSI can be a serious medical condition.

Steps can be taken to try to prevent, treat, and manage it, but you should not ignore it. Left untreated, the injury can become permanent.

RSI is the general term for a range of chronic musculoskeletal and nerve disorders in the hands, arms, shoulders, and neck. Because these injuries involve the body's connective tissue, pain and symptoms often travel. What may start out as a stiff neck can develop into a stiff neck and shoulders, or even a tingling in the fingers. That's why the specific diagnosis is so difficult to pinpoint. One skeptical British judge ruled that the symptoms were "too vague" to qualify as a medical condition. Clearly, he, like many other people, simply didn't understand it.

RSI goes by a number of other terms, including cumulative trauma disorder, occupational overuse syndrome, and repetitive motion disorder. All are labels for the same thing—a persistent and debilitating injury that in recent years has exploded in the workplace. These broad umbrella terms are used to cover a number of specific medical diagnoses, such as carpal tunnel syndrome, tennis elbow, and rotator cuff tendinitis. The labels—"repetitive strain," "cumulative trauma," "work-related upper-limb disorders," and "occupational overuse"—are all attempts to help explain the cause.

COSTS SOARING

There is some debate about the specific causes of these injuries, but there is no disagreement over the fact that RSI has become a significant problem in the workplace throughout the United States, Europe, Canada, Australia, and Japan. The U.S. Bureau of Labor Statistics reports roughly three hundred thousand cases of it a year, which amounts to nearly one-third of all injuries in the workplace. In 1981, RSI represented 18 percent of occupational illnesses; in 1995, it accounted for 63 percent, according to the BLS. At least half of all RSIs occur in offices.

The U.S. Labor Department estimates RSI costs employers twenty billion dollars a year in worker's compensation costs. That is one dollar of every three dollars spent on worker's compensation claims, a number that is expected to grow soon to half of every dollar spent on claims, according to the Occupational Safety and Health Administration. The total cost climbs to one hundred billion dollars, if the cost of lost workdays and retraining are figured in.

The problem of RSI is so significant that major universities and hospitals like Marquette University in Wisconsin and Mt. Sinai Hospital in New York have launched expensive studies into it, governments on all levels are pushing regulations to help prevent it, and both unions and employers have organized around it. Yet, despite the growing awareness of the problem, many experts believe that RSI is underreported. Many sufferers don't realize that their aches and pains might be caused by the work they are doing; others are reluctant to report their injuries, fearing reprisal by their employers.

Then there are people who don't show up as government statistics because they are working despite their injuries. One woman, a claims processor in New Jersey, lost feeling in her fingers. She had surgery and then returned to work but received a warning from management for making excessive errors. Despite the surgery, her hands had not returned to normal. Her supervisors told her to take more time to process claims, but that meant falling below her punishing quota of eight thousand keystrokes per hour.

Another woman had to have surgery on both wrists to relieve carpal tunnel syndrome. She returned to her job as a telephone service representative, taking phone orders at full speed. She worries, however, because her left hand sometimes still feels numb. "Should this recur, what do I do?" she asks.

"I'm a single mom. I have to work. Where do I go where there are no computers or typing?"

Both women fell into a bind many people with RSI face—their livelihood or their health. Many injured employees turn to worker's compensation, the system designed to protect employees in such a situation. But it is a safety net that is slow, frustrating, and confusing. Some people are afraid to file worker's compensation claims, fearing that it will stigmatize them. In addition, insurance companies and employers have made a push throughout the United States to make it tougher to receive worker's compensation. Companies say they need to reduce spiraling costs; unions say it's a way of rolling back benefits to workers.

AN OLD PROBLEM

RSI is not new. It was noted as early as 1717 by Bernandino Ramazzini, an Italian doctor regarded as the father of occupational medicine. He wrote of the "diseases of clerks and scribes," from "continuous sitting, repeated use of the hand, and strain of the mind." In 1864, a British medical journal reported similar complaints from milkmaids and shoemakers. And at the turn of the twentieth century, there were widespread reports of such injuries among British telegraph operators after the introduction of the Morse Code. Novelist Henry James had such a bad case of RSI that he had to turn to dictating his writing to secretaries.

In the 1950s and 1960s, RSI became a problem in Japan among keypunch operators. It burst into popular consciousness in the early 1980s in Australia, where an epidemic of injuries swept through the work force as offices and workplaces were computerized. The country's strong labor unions took up the issue and insisted on changes to protect workers, while prominent doctors insisted the injuries were psychosomatic. That insistence only fueled workers's anger and fanned the issue into a full-blown controversy in the nation's media. Some observers suggested that the RSI epidemic in Australia was a result of hysteria caused by the media. At the same time, scientists were doing serious research into the problem and finding that the roots of RSI were indeed physical.

RSI did not become widely known in the United States until the 1980s and 1990s, when increasing numbers of workers reported pain and weakness in their hands, arms, shoulders, and neck. That increase has been attributed, in part, to the growing computerization of the workplace. In 1980, only one in ten workers used computers on the job. Today, more than half do. Add to that the rapid spread of computers in the home and you have a lot of people spending a lot of time at computer keyboards. Experts like to talk about how the Internet is revolutionizing the global economy, but it is also revolutionizing the way many of us spend time at home. In addition, computerized technology allows people to work faster, harder, and with far less change in the pace and type of physical tasks to be done.

✖ OCCUPATIONAL HAZARDS

However, computers are not the only culprit. More sophisticated technology has enabled all kinds of workers to work faster and produce more. Assembly lines move much faster, and new machinery is used to do tasks once done by workers, resulting in what some academics call a *deskilling* of the work force, where workers do fewer and fewer skilled tasks. Many managers have heralded these changes as a boon to production, but the human cost is beginning to offset those gains. A growing number of doctors, physical and occupational therapists, and other medical professionals is sounding the warning: The human body was never meant to operate like a machine. As Rosa, an engraver who was forced to leave a job she loved because of RSI, says, "You could be made of the finest steel and you would break."

Technology is not the only culprit. Increasing competition in the global economy has forced companies to "downsize," laying off workers and combining jobs. In some cases it's cheaper to pay one worker overtime than it is to hire another worker. The pressure is to produce more with less. That means a work force anxious about job security and working harder to keep pace. That combination of job anxiety and increased workload, say some workers' advocates, is a recipe for RSI.

HUMAN TOLL

The human cost of RSI can be devastating. Rosa, who was fifty-six when she had to leave her job, moved to the United States when she was in her early twenties to marry the man she loved. Though she then spoke little English, she learned fast, worked hard, and made a life for herself. Rosa and her husband reared a family of four and later she took a job as a highly skilled engraver. She threw herself into it for fourteen years. "Work was like wings on my back," she says. "I didn't want to lose that."

One day, though, Rosa started to feel mysterious aches and pains in her arms and shoulders. She went from doctor to doctor and was told it was "all in my head." But it wasn't. The pain was so bad she couldn't hold her infant granddaughter, fearful she would drop her. Finally, she found a physical therapist who understood the problem and helped her. Though she has improved, Rosa is still unable to work. She has accepted that fact but still feels "a little core of anger," she says. "You give your soul to it . . . and you get the rug pulled out."

David, a graphic designer, started developing pains at the age of twenty-nine after just a few months of working long hours at his computer. He believes that his body was telling him to slow down. His wrist pain worries him, but after making some ergonomic adjustments to his equipment and learning to take regular breaks, he thinks he can manage it. Nonetheless, as a designer, he says, he is stunned that his state-of-the-art equipment was not designed to accommodate the human body. Though he believes he has his case under control, he knows a fellow graphic designer who has given up her job because of the pain in her hands.

RSI can happen to anyone, from pieceworkers to managers. It cuts across gender, age, race, income, and occupation. Even fairly young people are at risk. One of the factors associated with developing RSI is the length of time spent doing an injurious activity. That length of time is not measured in hours but in days, weeks, and months. For that reason, young people are less likely to get hurt than older people, who have spent more time doing such activities. But, according to the Bureau of Labor Statistics, more people ages fourteen to twenty-four are reporting injuries. Some therapists blame computers. Even toddlers use them, older children play video games on them, and more and more schools use them as part of their curriculum. In fact, a school that does not teach computer skills is likely to be regarded as woefully inadequate.

Before the explosion of RSI among office workers—once considered a low-risk occupation—it was prevalent enough among both meat cutters and musicians to prompt serious scientific studies. Although those seem like different occupations, there are similar risk factors in both—repetition, force, and awkward postures.

Guitarist Leo Kotke developed it from playing his instrument. In a 1987 interview with *Frets Magazine,* he described it this way: "I was halfway through a tune at a gig in Denver and suddenly my fingers wouldn't move. My whole arm froze up. It was like pushing a refrigerator across the floor. My doctor told me I had a problem with the sheathing on the tendons on my arm."

Kotke had to change his playing technique, getting rid of his finger picks and thumb pick. "I learned that you use everything in your whole arm to pick, not just your fingers," he said. "I found that I could play with less force and get more sound. . . . Now I have more dynamic range and a lot more different colors to draw on."

Concert pianist Leon Fleisher, a child prodigy from a Russian émigré family, developed RSI. It was crippling enough to send him to a succession of doctors and therapies and ultimately compel him to change his career and his life. "The gods hit you where it hurts," Fleisher said in a 1996 interview with the *Baltimore Sun.*

When Fleisher was afflicted at the height of his career in 1962, "it seemed as though one or another finger was a little bit lazy," he said. "The fingers weren't responding the way they always had. And my reaction was, 'I'm falling out of shape; I've got to work harder,' which, of course, is the wrong thing to do."

Three years later, his fourth and fifth fingers were curling into his palm. Within months Fleisher could no longer use his right hand to play piano. He felt despair, he said. "In a very real way, when this happened, I thought my life was over." He turned to teaching and developed a reputation as a masterful instructor. He began playing a left-handed repertoire. "And that really sustained me. Because I've made a career since 1983, a most unique career, out of five fingers," he said. Only recently has Fleisher begun—quietly, without publicity—playing a two-handed repertoire again.

Like Rosa and David, Kotke and Fleisher are people who had a lot to lose as a result of RSI. They were not malingerers, which some people with the injury have been accused of. In fact, scientific studies have found that this injury afflicts the hardest workers, not people who are trying to get out of work. Best-selling crime novelist Patricia Cornwell, who is known for her intensity about her work, told *Vanity Fair* magazine that she developed it after writing two hundred pages in ten days. Until J. Michael Straczynski, creator of the television show, "Babylon 5," bought an ergonomic keyboard, he had to stop typing every twenty minutes in order to ice his wrists, according to *Newsweek* magazine. People who don't want to work don't go to such lengths to work.

CLASH OVER CAUSE

Nor are people with RSI suffering from hysteria, or caught up in "media hype," as some observers have suggested. Some people who are worried about the proliferation of lawsuits against equipment manufacturers or the push for government regultion have tried to play down the seriousness of RSI. They say the science is "murky" and that little is known about its cause.

In fact, serious scientific research has investigated the cause, treatment, and management of RSI. The National Institute of Occupational Safety and Health has done several major studies into RSI, keyboards, and occupational risk factors. Currently, Johns Hopkins University, North Carolina State University, and the University of Wisconsin are conducting studies into RSI health concerns, job design, and equipment placement and design. The Communications Workers of America, which in the 1980s began noticing high rates of RSI among the telecommunications workers it represents, has pushed hard for these studies because union officials feel strongly that RSI health issues have not been addressed adequately.

Great strides have been made in applying ergonomics—the science of adapting tools and equipment to fit the human body—to the workplace. One sequin-factory owner who made ergonomic changes by providing his workers with adjustable chairs and redesigning a machine called a spooler saw his annual worker's compensation costs drop from ninety-seven thousand dollars in 1994 to forty-five hundred dollars in 1995. A Chrysler assembly plant that started a joint labor-management program reported an 80-percent drop in injuries requiring lost time from work. The 3M Company, after finding that more than half of its lost-time injuries among workers were due to RSI, instituted a sophisticated and aggressive ergonomics program in 1991. Five years later, cases of RSI had dropped by 58 percent. Other companies have had similar successes in reducing their costs—without having to spend a great deal of money on the ergonomic changes. Given that one worker's compensation claim can cost a business thousands of dollars, it makes sense to prevent RSI.

Just as important, numerous studies have documented gains in productivity after ergonomic changes were made. An Arthur D. Little Inc., 1996 survey of forty-five companies found that 70 percent of the companies surveyed reported increases in productivity after implementing ergonomics programs. At the same time, 30 percent reported improvements in product quality.

Despite those successes, some businesses have banded together to fight U.S. government regulation, fearing it would be too unwieldy, or costly, or simply because they oppose any regulation. However, unions, alarmed by the high numbers of workers affected by RSI, have rallied to push for an ergonomic standard to protect workers from ergonomic hazards. The issue is a serious one; at auto-assembly plants in Oklahoma

City, Oklahoma, and Dayton, Ohio, workers walked off the job or threatened strikes in part over complaints about ergonomics. They later won contract provisions that mandated improving ergonomic conditions. Those unions and others see this fight as a rallying cry. Few labor-management struggles have sparked the intensity of emotion in recent years.

PERSONAL COST

The reason for that intensity is simple: RSI can take an enormous toll not just financially but in human terms. Anyone who is forced out of work by an on-the-job injury faces profound insecurity—financial, professional, and personal. Most people with RSI are stricken in the prime of their lives, at a time when they are typically unprepared to confront the kind of upheaval brought by being forced out of work. Even those able to continue to work face insecurity because of their need to keep the injury under control. And the impact of RSI is compounded by the general lack of understanding of the problem. People with RSI don't look injured, even though the pain and injury it causes can be incapacitating.

People with RSI typically experience myriad emotions, ranging from denial and panic to anger. Sometimes they may seem volatile and self-absorbed; in reality, they are trying to make sense of an experience that doesn't seem to make sense. Most people are taught that if they work hard, they will get ahead—not be crippled. That isn't supposed to happen. Many RSI sufferers say they've coped by talking to others with the injury—either in formal support groups or through informal networks—because they are the people who truly understand it.

Physical pain is an unpleasant experience. When it persists, as it can with RSI, for days, weeks, or months, it has a profound effect on your outlook. It's hard to find the words to communicate to others what it's like, and it's even more unsettling to discover that most people don't want to hear about it.

Many people with RSI say they are shocked by the lack of support they encounter after being injured. They talk about feeling betrayed by bosses or coworkers who think they're malingering and a benefits system that forces them to prove they are not faking. Even more supportive friends and coworkers may make subtle suggestions that they are somehow physically "inferior" because they are injured.

Sometimes the impersonal nature of insurance companies and worker's compensation systems can be demoralizing. It is frustrating to see an injury that has affected almost every aspect of one's life be reduced to a number or form letter. One woman with RSI had been out of work for two years and was astonished to receive a letter from her disability insurance company telling her she was no longer disabled according to company guidelines and therefore no longer entitled to benefits. At the time, she was unable to do even simple household chores. Eventually, her doctor persuaded the company that she could not work, and her benefits were restored.

She was lucky. She had a doctor who was willing to be her advocate. Another woman who was fired because she could no longer work was stunned when a doctor told her that losing a job wasn't so bad for a woman. She surely would get married and not have to worry about it. Needless to say, she found another doctor.

The sexism she encountered was not unusual. Women with RSI often talk about having their complaints dismissed by doctors or managers as not being real, or if they are real, as not being serious enough to warrant attention. That problem is a reflection of the larger matter of women's health issues being ignored or downplayed by the medical establishment.

Although advocates of women's health issues have made great gains in recent years, sexism lingers. Add to that the fact that RSI is often associated with the workplace, where women have less clout and less earning power than men, and the issue becomes more highly charged.

Sexism is also an issue for men with RSI. Being able to take care of yourself and others is a trait closely intertwined with our notion of masculinity. A man who is physically unable to carry groceries—a task that may be out of reach for someone with RSI—is unlikely to elicit much sympathy. More likely, he would encounter outright scorn.

RSI strikes more women than men. Women suffer two out of three cases of RSI. People who have studied the injury attribute this to a variety of factors—smaller musculature and bone mass, hormonal changes, and the kinds of jobs women do that put them at greater risk. Being a woman, however, is not enough to put you a risk. Although the debate over what causes RSI continues, researchers have found certain risk factors, including poor workstation design, workload and pacing, general health, genetic predispositions, and activities outside work do contribute to the condition.

None of this is intended to suggest the victim is at fault. Companies eager to dodge liability try to say that; and in fact, that argument is often used as a defense in product-liability or worker's compensation lawsuits. To date, nearly all the product-liability suits filed against equipment manufacturers that have gone to trial have lost. Lawsuits filed by plaintiffs seeking worker's compensation for their RSI have had mixed results. Coverage of RSI by worker's compensation varies from state to state, but, as union advocates point out, workers who are refused worker's compensation are likely to end up in another system—the problem doesn't disappear. Instead, the burden is shifted.

❧

PREVENTING RSI

The key to dealing with the problem is prevention. Today people have the benefit of the experience of those who were injured before them; much of the equipment blamed for injuring people ten years ago has been taken off the market. Keyboard and workstation manufacturers have taken heed and are designing equipment with the needs of the human body in mind—in other words, ergonomic equipment. Injuries can be prevented or minimized if your workstation is set up with ergonomic considerations in mind. Often, changing a piece of equipment or making an adjustment in a workstation can make symptoms go away for people who have noted the symptoms early.

Many products being marketed today are labeled ergonomic; not all of them are. The most important feature of any ergonomic product is adjustability. People come in different shapes and sizes. You must be able to adjust the equipment to suit your needs. And, of course, if you don't bother to adjust it, it won't do you any good. Trained ergonomists can be helpful in setting up a safe, comfortable workstation. If you want to do it yourself, there are a number of considerations to keep in mind, but the most important thing is to avoid awkward, uncomfortable postures. Set up your workstation and get equipment that enables you to work comfortably, without straining.

Changing equipment and redesigning workstations may not be enough for some people. Jobs in which workers are compelled to work excessive overtime, are monitored electronically, or speed up at the end of a shift, when they are more likely to be fatigued, place people at high risk for RSI. Shifting the work load and rearranging work tasks can reduce that risk.

Ergonomic concerns are not limited to the workplace. Many people have hobbies or outside work that may contribute to an RSI problem. Many manufacturers have recognized this fact and have marketed products to address these concerns. For example, the Nevada Gaming Commission has approved the sale and distribution of ergonomically designed casino video games. The poker, blackjack, slot, and Keno video games are designed for greater comfort and less player fatigue, thus encouraging longer play and more profit for the casinos.

Whatever you do, be aware of the warning signs. It may be a seemingly unrelated headache that won't go away, a sense of heaviness or soreness in the arms, or an intermittent tingling in the fingers. The point is to pay attention to your body.

TREATING RSI

If you've missed the warning signs, don't blame yourself, because they're easy to miss. RSI is treatable. More and more doctors and therapists are beginning to understand it and treat it. Caught early, symptoms often disappear. Even if RSI is caught later, the symptoms usually can be brought under control. They may not disappear completely, and they may be something you will have to deal with for the rest of your life, but like many other conditions, the symptoms of RSI usually can be managed.

It's essential to get treatment as soon as you notice symptoms. The earlier you catch it, the better off you'll be. People who did not know what they had have been permanently injured, and, in some cases, crippled by RSI. This condition should be taken seriously.

One key to successful treatment is finding a doctor who is experienced, knowledgeable, caring, and on your side. You cannot do all the work that recovery entails on your own. Doctors and therapists are so immersed in the medical system that it's easy for them to forget that for most patients, being plunged into physical therapy and/or surgery can be a bewildering and frustrating experience. You need guidance. If you are confused, don't be afraid to ask questions.

Even more important than finding a good doctor is taking charge of your own recovery. A doctor and therapist can guide your recovery, but they cannot do it for you. Treat them as partners in your treatment. Setbacks will occur, but with time, they will happen less often. Recovery takes time and tenacity, but it can be an experience that changes your life in wonderful ways.

CHAPTER 2

WHAT EXACTLY IS RSI?

For Marion, it began after eighteen years of working as a secretary on Long Island. Every time she typed for long periods on her video display terminal, her right wrist and elbow would ache, and her pinkie would go numb. Initially, she ignored it. But over time, the pain worsened. It began to hit her hard when she came home from work. Her boss, who had heard about carpal tunnel syndrome, advised her to see a doctor.

Marion went to her family doctor, who was confused by her symptoms. Nonetheless, he prescribed splints and anti-inflammatory drugs. After ten days of that treatment, her pain had not abated. She went to another doctor, who also wasn't sure of the diagnosis. She began to feel frantic.

"Nobody could tell me, is it carpal tunnel? Is it not carpal tunnel? All I knew was that I was in pain, and nobody could tell me why," she says.

CONFUSION IS SO COMMON

Marion's experience is not uncommon. Despite the prevalence of RSI and publicity associated with it, many physicians—even specialists—are unfamiliar with its various manifestations. One reason may be the medical literature on the subject; there is no consistent diagnosis, etiology, prognosis, or name for the disorder. And just what causes RSI has become a controversial issue; labeling the condition as work-related or non-work-related can determine how the bills are paid. Not every doctor wants to step into that quagmire. And, in fact, it is hard for many people to believe that a seemingly harmless activity such as typing on a computer keyboard could cause so much damage.

Misdiagnosis happens more often than medical professionals like to admit, say experts and sufferers alike. Paul Taylor, a medical reporter for the Toronto *Globe* and *Mail* wrote about his own experience with RSI in a December 27, 1993, article: "It is not so unusual for patients to be misdiagnosed. I have talked to patients who, on the advice of their doctors, underwent rib removal, breast reduction, or the stripping away of nerves—only to have the pain and numbness continue."

If a doctor says there is nothing wrong, get a second opinion. RSI can be a serious condition and should not be left untreated. More likely, if a doctor is confused by the diagnosis, he may refer you to a specialist in neurology, orthopedics, or rehabilitation medicine.

As the number of cases grows, scientists and medical professionals are beginning to understand the various conditions labeled RSI. Carpal tunnel syndrome is the most commonly known type, but there are many others that can be just as debilitating. Although each condition has distinct symptoms, pain and swelling are usually associated with all of them. It's the body's way of protecting itself by trying to force you to rest. In addition, it is not unusual for a patient to have more than one of these RSIs.

The basic mechanism of injury is fairly simple: When you curl your finger, a muscle in the arm pulls a tendon that runs through the wrist into the hand. In effect, the tendon is like a long pulley controlling movement in the finger. The more you repeat the action, the more the tendon is stressed. If your arm or hand is forced into awkward positions, the more the tendon is stressed. Over time, injury can result.

Tendons and ligaments are a type of connective tissue called fascia, a weblike, durable sheath that connects muscle to bone. For any movement to happen, muscles on one side of a joint contract, and muscles on the other side must lengthen, or release. If an injury occurs, the fascia actually undergoes a chemical change, becoming thicker and tougher. To protect the body, the fascia will tighten up and begin sticking muscle to muscle, or muscle to nerve, or nerve to ligament, etc. Movement is likely to be less fluid. If scar tissue forms, movement may be further impeded.

Although many people think of RSI as an injury solely to the hands and arms, many cases involve the neck as well, says Jackie Ross, a Manhattan-based physical therapist who has treated many cases of RSI. You may, for example, feel symptoms in your hands and arms because of a nerve that is compressed in the neck. People tend to think of body parts as separate elements, which they are, but they are connected by extensive pathways that run throughout the body. Once a nerve is affected, it can cause problems all along its path, all the way down to the fingertips. For that reason, Ross says, it's important to look at a patient's posture. (Posture will be discussed in greater detail in later chapters.)

Some doctors and physical therapists believe that RSI usually begins in the back and then progresses to the neck, arms, and hands. Often, patients seek treatment for pain in their hands and arms; but when questioned, they remember the pain beginning in their back and shoulders. A pair of mid-back muscles, the upper and lower trapezius, holds the torso and shoulders in place. If forced into the same position for long periods of time, as when you are working at a computer keyboard, those muscles become exhausted. Though it doesn't seem like much physical exertion, it does take a great deal of effort to hold the body in place. When the principal muscles for a task stop working, the body relies on others that aren't designed for the task. Pain and injury can result.

People develop different injuries, even though all are grouped under the category of RSI, because each person's body has different areas of weakness and strength. This chapter will discuss the better-known and most common diagnoses of RSI. It is meant merely as a guideline. Do not self-diagnose. Individual diagnoses vary. Always consult with a doctor.

❧ NERVE DISORDERS

Carpal Tunnel Syndrome

Most people have heard of carpal tunnel syndrome. In fact, they frequently misuse the term when talking about any of the hand, arm, and shoulder problems they associate with typing on video display terminals. It was what Marion thought of when her arms and hands began to hurt. She did, in fact, have carpal tunnel syndrome.

Carpal tunnel syndrome is a fairly simple problem. Inside the wrist is a carpal tunnel formed by bone and tough ligament. A bundle of nine tendons of the forearm and the median nerve passes through it to the hand. The median nerve conducts brain impulses to the thumb, forefinger, middle finger, and half of the ring finger. Excessive up-and-down motions of the wrist—which can occur during typing—can cause swelling of the carpal tunnel lining. That, in turn, can cause compression of the median nerve.

Medical professionals point out that "true" carpal tunnel syndrome is not as common as people think. You may be experiencing symptoms of it as a result of tendinitis, for example. Or, as Ross points out, the median nerve can be compressed at any point as it runs from the neck to the wrist, causing symptoms. A series of specific diagnostic tests (discussed in more detail in chapter 6) can determine whether you have true carpal tunnel syndrome.

Repetitive motions are not the only cause of carpal tunnel syndrome. Researchers have found it to be associated with pregnancy, the use of oral contraceptives, diabetes, thyroid disease, menopause, and acute trauma. Smoking, drinking, and consuming caffeine may also be factors. A 1996 study reported in the *Journal of Occupational Medicine* found that the use of tobacco, caffeine, and alcohol slows down the brain impulses passing through the median nerve. Researchers compared workers with carpal tunnel syndrome with those without symptoms, and found that those with symptoms smoked more, consumed slightly more caffeine, and had a greater history of alcohol abuse. The study concluded that those drugs affected median nerve slowing, but also said the effects of the drugs explained only a small portion of the total risk. In other words, while they may be contributing factors, they are not likely to be the sole cause.

In fact, carpal tunnel syndrome has been widely reported in a number of occupations—carpentry, journalism, administrative work, supermarket cashiering, ditchdigging, surgery, assembly-line work, knitting, and other careers that call on wrists to work in a repetitive or forceful manner. In the past, it was called "stitcher's wrist" and "cotton-twister's hand." With the onset of video games, it has earned a new name—"Space Invader's wrist," according to the U.S. Department of Health and Human Services.

When the median nerve is compressed, sufferers report feeling tingling and pain in their hands, primarily in the index and middle fingers and part of the ring finger. Symptoms are felt in the palmar side of the hand. Gradually, the pain grows worse, causing night waking. The night wakefulness occurs because most people sleep with their wrists bent, a position that exacerbates symptoms of carpal tunnel syndrome. Other symptoms may include shooting pains up the arm and a feeling of swelling in the fingers, even though no swelling is visible. The symptoms often come and go, so it is not uncommon for a sufferer to dismiss it as nothing serious at first.

However, left untreated, the condition worsens. You may detect changes in fingertip sensation. Grip strength diminishes; you may find yourself dropping objects. A neurologist reported in a medical newsletter that he and his colleagues had treated several people in the emergency room with scald burns on the front of their thighs. In each case, the patient had picked up a coffeepot and then dropped it. The underlying cause in each case was carpal tunnel syndrome. In a separate incident, a librarian afflicted with carpal tunnel syndrome recalled with horror the day she dropped her fifteen-month-old baby.

The symptoms can be frightening. Because carpal tunnel syndrome is not uncommon, it's easy for others to minimize the experience. But the human hand is, of course, essential to performing tasks that render us human. Losing the use of it to any degree is serious, indeed.

Fortunately, losing the full use of a hand happens rarely. Carpal tunnel syndrome is a gradual condition, occurring over a period of years. And many medical professionals are familiar enough with it to intervene early and effectively. Often, surgery is recommended. While some professionals believe that surgery has been overused, at least one study found that complications from surgery are uncommon. More on the treatment of carpal tunnel syndrome and other conditions detailed here will be discussed in chapters 6, 7, and 8. (See Figure 2.1.)

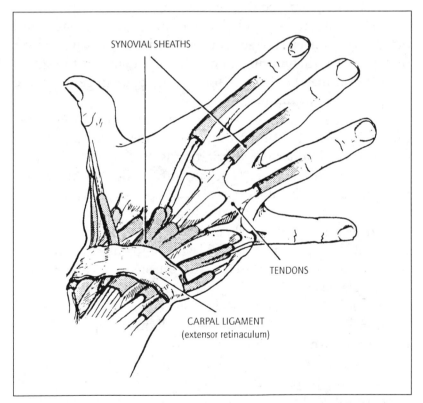

SYNOVIAL SHEATHS

TENDONS

CARPAL LIGAMENT
(extensor retinaculum)

FIGURE 2.1: A pictorial view of the finger tendons, their sheaths, and the carpal ligament in the hand.

Reprinted from "Cumulative Trauma Disorders," 1988 publication of The National Institute for Occupational Safety and Health.

Ulnar Nerve Irritation

For most people, the ulnar nerve is better known as the "funny bone." The shooting pain that comes when one hits that spot in their elbow is painfully familiar. That's the same kind of pain that results from an irritated ulnar nerve, which is a terminal branch of a network of nerves originating in the neck. One journalist suffering from ulnar-nerve irritation described it as "like being plugged into an electrical outlet."

The ulnar nerve supplies sensation to the little finger and half the ring finger, so when it is irritated, it is not uncommon to experience tingling in the hand, particularly in those fingers. It also may be difficult to separate your fingers. Muscle atrophy is not uncommon.

Generally, the cause is repetitive motion or activity that puts continuous pressure on the nerve. One particular activity associated with ulnar-nerve irritation is leaning on your elbow while you work or drive. That cuts off the flow of blood and puts pressure on the ulnar nerve. In all RSIs, good circulation is important. Muscles normally produce metabolic wastes that are carried away in the blood when it flows freely. When circulation is restricted, that flushing of the wastes, or toxins, stops. Instead, they accumulate in the muscle tissue, causing aches and fatigue.

A related condition is cubital tunnel syndrome, where the ulnar nerve is entrapped at the elbow. The cubital tunnel is located in the funny bone area of the elbow. Symptoms of cubital tunnel syndrome include numbness on the inside of the hand, tingling in the ring and little fingers, and loss of sensation. The forearm muscles may be painful, and pain may travel downward from the elbow to the little finger. Flexing of the forearm may cause pain as well. If the syndrome progresses untreated, atrophy of the muscle pad below the little finger may develop.

This condition is found in people who engage in activities that require repeated bending and straightening of their elbows, such as pulling levers on a machine, or who rest their elbows on hard surfaces. It used to be called "telephone operator's elbow" because telephone operators used to rest their elbows on a hard bench while switching telephone lines. It can also be caused by a direct blow or injury to the elbow. It also has been diagnosed in musicians, particularly guitarists.

When conservative treatments fail for cubital tunnel syndrome, surgery is sometimes recommended in order to prevent permanent nerve damage. The most common operation performed for cubital tunnel syndrome actually involves moving the ulnar nerve from behind the bump of the elbow bone (medial epicondyle) to the front, which gives the nerve some slack when the elbow is bent.

Radial Tunnel Syndrome

Radial tunnel syndrome is considered relatively rare, though some researchers believe it is largely unrecognized because its symptoms are easily confused with those of tennis elbow or tenosynovitis. You may be at risk for radial tunnel syndrome if you do work that involves twisting your arm faceup and facedown frequently and forcefully.

In radial tunnel syndrome, one has pain on both sides of the forearms. Sufferers find it hard to make a fist. Twisting motions can be excruciating. Weakness and a loss of sensation may occur on the top side of the hand, although numbness doesn't usually occur. A recent study conducted in the United Kingdom recommends that physicians consider the possibility of radial tunnel syndrome in patients who have forearm and wrist pain that does not respond to conventional treatment.

Nerve entrapment is associated with radial tunnel syndrome more often than previously thought. Compression of the nerve occurs when you, for example, drape your arm over the back of a chair. Though no particular occupation has been identified as being prone to radial tunnel syndrome, carpenters are an example of a group at risk because they have to twist their elbows and may need to lean on an arm to accomplish a task. In addition, certain underlying conditions, such as diabetes mellitus, may make some patients more susceptible to nerve entrapments.

In extreme cases, surgery is recommended.

TENDON DISORDERS

Tendons are ropelike bands that connect muscle to bone. They transfer force from muscle to bone when you move your hands, arms, and fingers. Generally, it is the large muscle groups that bear the load for heavier work; tendons are responsible for fine-motor functions, such as writing, typing, sewing, and similar activities.

Much fine-motor work, such as office work, involves static postures. If you work at a computer, for example, you'll probably pause fairly often to compose a thought, find a key, or figure out a function. While pausing, you probably are holding your arms in a bent position, perhaps resting your hands on the keyboard or a wrist rest. That is considered a static posture because although you are resting your arms, the muscles are still contracting to hold the arms in the bent position.

When muscles are in a fairly continual state of contraction, a condition known as "static muscle loading" occurs. Because the muscles are contracted—but not regularly relaxed—circulation is decreased and waste products are not removed from the blood as quickly as they should be. That leads to muscle soreness.

Many people are accustomed to muscle soreness and may be inclined to ignore it, especially if they don't understand the cause. Prolonged muscle soreness without relief may lead to more serious tendon disorders.

Tendinitis

Most people think of tendinitis as a benign condition. They've heard of athletes who have it but still play. In fact, racquet sports and throwing have been associated with it. Generally, tendinitis is not an overly serious condition. But it can be painful and debilitating. One man with a severe case described it as feeling like "metal scraping against metal."

Tendinitis occurs when a tendon is tensed over and over, so much so that it initially becomes inflamed. A healthy tendon is smooth. One that is damaged can fray or break apart; it becomes thick and bumpy.

Sufferers report feeling a dull, aching pain and heaviness in the affected area. Because these tendons are constantly in use, the injury can be slow to heal. Rest is important. Without it, the tendon may be permanently damaged.

When the condition becomes chronic, it is considered a tendinosis, a degenerative, painful condition occurring as a result of microtears. These are tiny tears in the tendons, and microscarring, or tiny scar tissue, caused by overuse.

Tenosynovitis

Tenosynovitis and tendinitis usually occur simultaneously. Tenosynovitis is the inflammation of the fluid-filled sheath—

called the synovium—that surrounds the tendon. When the tendon is repeatedly tensed, to protect it the sheath produces more fluid. However, excessive fluid causes the sheath to become swollen and painful. This condition can cause nerve compression, most commonly within the carpal tunnel, which might lead to initial confusion about the diagnosis.

Symptoms of tenosynovitis include stiffness and pain that can range from dull and aching to burning. People with tenosynovitis may also experience swelling and crepitus, which is a clicking or cracking noise sometimes made by moving a joint.

Simple tasks become impossible. A Los Angeles journalist recalls the day she asked a coworker to cut the potatoes in the beef stew she had for lunch because she couldn't do it herself. On another day, her husband found her reduced to tears in their laundry room because she was unable to fold the wash.

Sufferers also frequently report being affected by changes in barometric pressure. Some medical professionals believe that joint pressure may be altered by changes in barometric pressure, although there is nothing specific in the scientific literature that addresses this.

Women with acute cases of tenosynovitis report worse symptoms just before their menstrual period.

Repeated movements of the wrist and forcefully extending the hand to either side are activities associated with tenosynovitis. It also can be caused by infection.

Stenosing Tenosynovitis

Stenosing tenosynovitis is the progressive restriction of the sheath surrounding the tendon. At this point, the condition is chronic. Two common diagnoses fall into this category: De Quervain's disease and trigger finger.

De Quervain's disease, named for Swiss surgeon Fritz De Quervain who first identified it in 1895, affects the tendons at the base of the thumb that are used to pull the thumb away from the hand. The tendons glide back and forth through the synovial lining, which can become inflamed, causing friction when the tendons move. Symptoms include acute pain at the base of the thumb, which may radiate to the hand or even the forearm. A simple task like holding a pen can be difficult, or even impossible.

One cause is frequent extension and flexion of the wrist. Extension is when you bend your wrist up and back; flexion is when you bend your wrist down toward the palm. De Quervain's disease has been documented in a number of occupations—punch-press operators, sewers, and cutters—that require the repeated movement and ulnar deviation of the wrist, which is bending the wrist toward the little finger.

Rapid rotation of the wrist—the movement used to hit a space bar on a computer keyboard, for example—is also associated with the disease. Other motions of the wrist and hand associated with it are wringing, grasping, turning, and twisting.

Another type of stenosing tenosynovitis is trigger finger. In this condition, the sheath surrounding the tendon becomes swollen and restricts movement of the tendon in the finger, making it difficult to straighten it after it is bent. Or, a nodule or bump on the tendon sheath impedes tendon movement.

In mild cases, the sufferer experiences resistance or catching when trying to extend the fingers after making a fist. The affected finger will be tender and make a soft, crackling sound whenever you attempt to move it. In more advanced cases, the finger locks in a bent position. It can be painful, and any attempt to straighten it out will cause a snapping or jerking movement. Swelling may also be present.

In an extreme case, the patient may be able to extend the finger only by pulling it with the other hand. Or, the finger may become locked into position and cannot be moved at all.

For many people with trigger finger, the symptoms are worse first thing in the morning because blood may accumulate in tissues during sleep. And because most people sleep with their hands flexed, swelling may occur. Finger movement becomes easier after waking because physical activity encourages the movement of pooled fluid out of tissues.

Trigger finger is associated with forcefully using tools that have hard or sharp edges, or one that has a handle too large for the hand. It also occurs when any finger other than the thumb is repeatedly flexed against pressure.

Surgery to open the tendon sheath is performed in cases where the patient has excessive pain and loss of functional ability.

Ganglion Cyst

A ganglion cyst is one of the few obviously visible RSIs. It is a small bump or bumps, generally on the back of the hand or wrist located at a joint capsule or tendon sheath. It occurs when fluid gathers in a puddle and causes the synovial sheath to swell. A cyst can come and go and often can be left untreated because it is usually benign. The size of the cyst may increase or decrease, depending upon how much the patient uses his hand.

Anyone who has ever had a ganglion cyst probably has been given unsolicited advice on how to treat it: Smash it with a heavy book (hence the term *Bible bump*).

That is not advisable, however. A ganglion cyst can be associated with nerve compression—ganglions can occur within the carpal tunnel—and cause shooting pains in the arm. In an extreme case, surgery may be warranted. Smashing it with a book is not. When the ganglion is not painful, surgery is done only for cosmetic reasons.

Tennis Elbow (Epicondylitis)

Tennis elbow is manifested by pain and swelling at the point where tendons join bone at the elbow. The extensor tendon that is attached to the elbow controls the movements of the hand and wrist. When it becomes irritated and inflamed, pain radiates down the arm and is felt on the outside or inside of the elbow. Medial epicondylitis, or *pitcher's elbow*, is an inflammation of the tendons leading to the wrist and finger flexors. The term *epicondylitis* refers to the epicondyles, which are the two bony bumps found at the lower corners of the humerus bone at the elbow.

Tennis elbow is so named because it can occur when you hit a backhand shot in tennis. The elbow straightens and the wrist extends as you strike the ball. Done repeatedly, if the racquet grip is too narrow, those motions require increased tension by the muscles to hold the racquet. Microtears in muscle and tendon can result because the flexors are contracting to hold the racquet while the extensors are firing to hit the backhand.

However, most people who get tennis elbow have not played the game—at least not regularly—for years. The same combination of lengthening and contracting can occur while sitting at a keyboard and typing. And when muscle and tendon are subjected to repeated microtears, tendinitis occurs. Usually, the tendon tears in a V shape, which makes healing harder.

Well-known among athletes, tennis elbow is also being found increasingly among musicians and journalists.

Rotator Cuff Tendinitis

The rotator cuff is a group of tendons and muscles that provides the shoulder with mobility and stability. Symptoms include a sharp, localized pain, and a significant lessening of mobility. A person with rotator cuff tendinitis finds overhead movements difficult and experiences stiffness and weakness. He may also feel a catching when using the arm.

Bursitis, an inflammation of the bursa, the protective cushion around the rotator cuff, may be diagnosed with rotator cuff tendinitis. The bursa, which is a fluid-filled sac rather like the rosin bag a baseball pitcher uses, protects areas of the body such as the shoulder, knee, and elbow where repeated pressure is exerted during movement. There are two bursa, one that interfaces with the rotator cuff tendon and one under the deltoid muscle. A tendon that is frayed or inflamed from overuse in turn irritates the adjacent bursa, causing bursitis. This is a painful condition that can limit shoulder mobility.

Occupational health studies have shown that bursitis is caused by work that places the elbows in an elevated position which puts pressure on the shoulders. Impingement of the rotator cuff tendon under one of the shoulder ligaments occurs when you lift your arm overhead. Because bursitis is associated with frequent overhead reaching, try to limit your reaching or do it in a way so that the arms are not extended more than thirty degrees away from your body.

This can progress from an acute to chronic condition. Acute bursitis may begin with a dull pain that becomes more intense and then travels down the arm. Moving the arm is painful; so is trying to lie down on that shoulder. When bursitis is chronic, the pain is milder but much longer-term. You probably feel it only when lifting your arm above shoulder height. But other problems may result from chronic bursitis: bone spurs, which can impinge the rotator cuff tendon; muscle atrophy; and ruptures of the tendon can result, usually in people older than forty. In addition, the distal (or distant) segment of the rotator cuff has poor blood supply, and healing is difficult.

❉

NEUROVASCULAR DISORDERS

Thoracic Outlet Syndrome

Thoracic outlet syndrome is a general term for the compression of the nerves and blood vessels between the neck and shoulder. When such a compression occurs, circulation to the area is impeded, thus depriving the muscles and tendons of essential nutrients and slowing the removal of toxins.

It can cause pain and tingling in the neck, shoulder, arm, and hand. Because of the tingling and the fact that, like carpal tunnel syndrome, it is more common among women, it is sometimes mistaken for carpal tunnel syndrome.

Sufferers also report feeling coldness and weakness in their fingers, hand, and forearm. Overhead reaches can be painful and cause tingling as well.

People with posture that impedes circulation, such as rounded shoulders, are vulnerable to thoracic outlet syndrome. Occupational health studies have found it among mail carriers who carry heavy shoulder bags. In fact, anyone experiencing symptoms of thoracic outlet syndrome probably should avoid carrying heavy bags or knapsacks. Typically, there is tightness of the chest muscles (pectoralis minor muscles), so that when a knapsack is worn, it pulls the muscles tight against the neurovascular supply and causes symptoms. Treatment focuses on stretching the pectoralis minor muscles.

Thoracic outlet syndrome can also be caused by certain chronic diseases and congenital defects, such as an extra rib. It is important to rule out cervical rib tumors. At least one study has found that poor outcome of treatment is related to obesity.

Raynaud's Disease

In Raynaud's disease, the blood vessels are constricted, causing fingers to become cold and pale. The paleness may be followed by a bluish tinge and then redness. Pain and numbness may accompany the changes in coloration. It can lead to the eventual loss of sensation in the hands, and a loss of control. Later symptoms include chronic infections around the fingernails.

Primary Raynaud's has no known cause. Secondary Raynaud's, the type that is considered a Repetitive Strain Injury, has several causes. Occupational health studies have found it to be associated with the use of vibrating tools, like jackhammers, and with typing. It is also associated with rheumatoid arthritis, thoracic outlet syndrome, and lupus. It occurs in men and women, although it is more common in women younger than forty.

Because smoking causes blood vessels to constrict, it is unwise to smoke if you have been diagnosed with Raynaud's disease. In fact, it's best to avoid any exposure to cigarette smoke. In addition, certain medications can trigger it.

Typically, warmth relieves symptoms. Avoiding exposure to cold in any form is advisable.

OTHER RELATED DISORDERS

Myofascial Pain Syndrome and Fibromyalgia

Myofascial pain syndrome is the diffuse pain and stiffness felt deep in the muscle tissues. The fasciae are membranes of varying thicknesses and strengths that surround the muscles; their primary function is to cover and protect the muscles. With myofascial pain syndrome, the fasciae get tight and impede the muscles from stretching. Muscles need to be able to stretch and relax in order to promote good blood flow and thus receive the necessary nutrients. Myofascial pain prevents this, and painful trigger spots, or painful nodules, can develop. When a trigger spot is touched, the pain can be exquisite and often will travel out from that spot to another part of the body. This is called referred pain. For example, if you have a trigger spot in your neck, you may well feel referred pain in your head, shoulder, upper back, and/or hand.

Fibromyalgia, by contrast, is a systemic form of myofascial pain. Strictly speaking, fibromyalgia may not always be an RSI. Its cause is unknown, although it is associated with people who have abnormal sleep patterns and immune system changes that resemble those caused by a chronic infection. Often, it is confused with carpal tunnel syndrome. It is included here because some researchers argue that when the fibromyalgia consists of pain localized in one part of the body, it is caused by repetitive motions. Fibromyalgia consists of tender points—not necessarily in muscle—that can also occur over bone. A recent survey looking at fibromyalgia and its relation to work activities found that typing, prolonged sitting and/or standing, stress, and heavy lifting or bending exacerbate the condition.

Symptoms include severe aching, excessive fatigue, swelling of the extremities, and numbness and tingling. You may wake up feeling stiff and exhausted, even though you've had plenty of sleep. Fibromyalgia can be debilitating, necessitating hospitalization in some cases. The most important symptom for most patients is pain, and studies show that fibromyalgia patients have an abnormally heightened pain reaction, which may indicate a biochemical connection. The onset varies. Some patients say it just crept up on them; others point to a trigger, such as an illness or accident. Doctors don't understand why different types of triggers seem to precipitate it.

Fibromyalgia is more common among women. Recent research appears to have debunked the notion that it is caused by depression, although any chronic pain condition is generally related to some degree of depression. However, because doctors often find it difficult to diagnose due to the apparent lack of objective physical findings, it has been suggested that fibromyalgia is psychosomatic. It is not. Some patients have been given a diagnosis of "psychogenic rheumatism," which implies it is all in the mind. The pain is in your muscles, not your mind.

Writer's Cramp (Focal Dystonia)

Although there are different types of dystonias, or movement disorders, in the body, the term *focal dystonia* indicates that the symptoms are localized in one part of the body. The type of focal dystonia that is considered an RSI is writer's cramp. Most people have experienced it momentarily at one time or another, but someone suffering from true writer's cramp experiences involuntary cramping and eventually loses some control over the hand. This type of dystonia affects the muscles of the hand and sometimes the forearm, and occurs during handwriting. It is also known as typist's cramp, pianist's cramp, musician's cramp, and golfer's cramp.

An early symptom is a deterioration in your handwriting. Focal dystonias have been diagnosed among musicians. Scientists are currently studying a range of dystonias and, in particular, are looking at the abnormal patterns of muscle actions that occur with dystonias. (See Table 2.1.)

TABLE 2.1: CONDITIONS AND SYMPTOMS

CONDITION	SYMPTOM
Carpal tunnel syndrome	Tingling and pain in hands, primarily in the index and middle fingers and part of the ring finger. Shooting pains up the arm; sometimes night waking caused by pain. Possible feeling of swelling in the fingers. Grip problems.
Ulnar-nerve irritation	Tingling in the hand, primarily in the fourth and fifth fingers. May be hard to separate the fingers. Muscle atrophy common.
Cubital tunnel syndrome	Tingling, numbness, loss of sensation, and muscle atrophy.
Radial tunnel syndrome	Pain on both sides of the forearms. Twisting motions and making a fist difficult. Possible weakness and loss of sensation on top side of hand, although numbness doesn't usually occur.
Tendinitis	Dull, aching pain. Feeling of heaviness in affected area.
Tenosynovitis	Stiffness. Pain ranging from dull to burning. Possible swelling and crepitus.
De Quervain's disease	Acute pain at base of thumb that may radiate to hand or forearm. Grip difficult.
Trigger finger	Difficulty making a fist or straightening fingers. May hear crackling or snapping when straightening attempted. Possible swelling. Pain present.
Ganglion cyst	Visible swelling in the form of a bump or bumps, usually on the back of the hand. Usually not exceptionally painful.
Tennis elbow	Radiating pain, felt on outside or inside of elbow.

Table continued overleaf

TABLE 2.1: CONDITIONS AND SYMPTOMS, *continued*

CONDITION	SYMPTOM
Rotator cuff tendinitis	Sharp, localized pain. Range of motion restricted. Overhead movements difficult. Stiffness and weakness present.
Bursitis	Pain ranging from dull to burning. Possible muscle atrophy.
Thoracic outlet syndrome	Pain and tingling in the neck, shoulder, arm, and hand. Coldness and weakness in fingers, hand, and forearm. Overhead reaches may cause pain and tingling. Difficult to feel pulse.
Raynaud's disease	Coldness and paleness in fingers. Possible loss of sensation in hands, eventual loss of control of hands.
Myofascial pain syndrome	Painful trigger spots that radiate pain when pressed.
Fibromyalgia	Severe aching. Numbness, tingling, and swelling. Excessive fatigue. Sleep disturbances.
Writer's cramp	Involuntary cramping of the hand.

❀
DON'T DIAGNOSE YOURSELF

The myriad technical terms and diagnoses can be overwhelming. As a consumer, knowledge is your best weapon. Although it is never advisable to diagnose yourself, it's important to know what questions to ask about your particular condition.

Stephanie, a California educator who suffers from work-related carpal tunnel syndrome and tendinitis, says, "Like a lot of people, I didn't recognize what the symptoms meant."

One writer in the Midwest remembers fearing he had multiple sclerosis the first time he felt the throbbing aches on the top of his hands, stabs of pain in his wrists, and numbness in his thumbs and index fingers. He even pulled out medical books and read about the progression of multiple sclerosis. His doctor tested him for it, along with a variety of other diseases, but didn't find anything. The writer finally made the connection to RSI himself when he realized that he was experiencing the pain after typing on his keyboard.

After what he calls *pilgrimages* to specialists near his home and out of state, "it dawned on me that doctors didn't have a clue." But with rest, exercise, and a concerted effort to learn about RSI, he has succeeded in managing his injury. Today, years after his initial injury, he doesn't even remember the exact diagnosis he was eventually given.

More and more doctors are becoming familiar with RSI and its treatment. It is particularly important that they listen, take an appropriate work history, and review all activities the patient may be performing that are repetitive in nature. Treatment options will be discussed in chapters 8 and 9. But as is true with any medical condition, it is important for you to take charge of your health. Remember: It's your body.

CHAPTER 3

WHAT CAUSES RSI?

❧

*Eileen, a data entry operator at an insurance com-
pany, thought she must have done something horribly
wrong when her arms started to burn. She went to
a doctor, who did a series of tests, but could find
nothing. He suggested the problem was in her head.*

*The burning persisted. Her job consisted of typ-
ing eight hours a day. The data entry operators in her
group got few breaks; anyone who wanted to use the
bathroom had to raise her hand and get permission
from the supervisor. Their keystrokes were electronically monitored, and an operator who did not meet
the standards set by the company could lose her job.*

*It was a grueling routine, and Eileen hated it.
But she needed the job to support herself and her
teenage daughter. Lately, she had become careless
about her diet, eating junk food and not exercising. It
was hard to get motivated to do anything because she
was so exhausted when she came home. And, now, her
arms hurt—a lot.*

"When the doctor said it was in my head, I really thought I was crazy," she recalls.

Ironically, she went to see a psychotherapist, who had heard of RSI, and sent her to another doctor. There, she learned she was suffering from severe, work-related tenosynovitis.

"I was so mad when I found out!" she says. "I had been thinking all along that this was my fault, that I had done something wrong, I hadn't been eating right, that I was drinking too much, and then the first doctor I saw told me I was crazy. And then I find out that it wasn't in my head, it was in my arms, and that it wasn't my fault!"

IT'S NOT YOUR FAULT

Probably the most important thing to remember in understanding the causes of RSI is that it is not your fault.

RSI has sneaked up on a generation of workers and the medical and scientific communities. When the advances of technology were first trumpeted in the workplace, few people ever thought they could cause physical problems in workers. Some people still have difficulty believing it—whether it's a doctor who has never seen RSI before or an employer wary of worker's compensation costs or even legal liability.

Just what causes RSI has been the subject of heated debate, as injured workers have sued equipment manufacturers and as business and government have clashed over regulations aimed at preventing it in the workplace.

Unfortunately, the answer isn't simple.

It is wrong to blame the victims of RSI when the scientific and medical communities cannot provide all the answers.

RSI and its causes are the subject of ongoing research at the National Institute of Occupational Safety and Health, Mt. Sinai Hospital in New York, and several universities. So far, researchers—many of whom have been guided by the reports of people with RSI—have found some important clues The physiological mechanisms of RSI are not well understood, but they probably include the depletion of needed oxygen to tissues; the lack of lubricating fluids for tendons; the buildup of toxins in the tissues; and changes in metabolism. These have been linked to a number of factors:

- posture and positioning
- repetition
- force
- duration
- vibration
- workstation and equipment design
- job design (including work load and pace of work)
- stress

All of these factors will be discussed in this chapter. Because they are often interrelated, it's important to consider each one when trying to understand what causes RSI.

Again, it's important to remember that it's not your fault.

❈
POSTURE AND POSITIONING

Despite the name "Repetitive Strain Injury," researchers have found posture to be one of the most significant factors causing RSI. This is a deceptive problem because poor posture often feels comfortable. Bad equipment or workstation design can force you into awkward postures, whether you work on an assembly line or at a computer keyboard. And no one's body will perform well from a weak or unstable posture or a strained position.

Perhaps the best advice on posture is not to sit upright in a rigid pose but to try to keep your body balanced. More on how to achieve good posture will be discussed in chapter 5.

Static Muscle Loading

The human body is designed for movement. You can test that notion yourself by recalling how quickly you feel tired after standing still for a few minutes, as opposed to walking.

Muscles in a dynamic activity contract and relax rhythmically and receive an adequate blood supply. By contrast, muscles forced into a static position—extending the arms for a long period of time while typing, for example—don't perform rhythmic contracting and relaxing. Instead, in contracting continuously, they miss the cycle of relaxation that brings a supply of fresh, oxygenated blood to the tissues. Soreness can result.

Many jobs, particularly office and manufacturing jobs that involve piecework, don't permit much freedom of movement. Instead, the body is forced into static postures for long periods of time. This leads to a condition called "static muscle loading." Researchers, particularly in Australia, have linked static muscle loading to RSI. It can happen while typing or working at a sewing machine, among other things.

It's problematic because you don't feel anything going wrong while doing it; but static muscle loading over a long period of time can cause serious injury. Some researchers believe that muscles subjected to repeated static muscle loading actually adapt by shortening themselves with fibrous tissue so that they don't have to contract. That forces tendons to stretch, something they're not designed to do, which can lead to tissue damage.

Static muscle loading can be avoided by making ergonomic changes to a workstation, taking frequent breaks,
and stretching. (This will be discussed in greater detail in
chapters 5 and 10.)

Posture Imbalance

Most people deviate from what is considered perfect balance.
Minor misalignments are not a problem. Major imbalances
are. That's when muscle strains occur. Just as improperly
aligned tires on a car show uneven wear and tear, muscles that
are out of balance have more wear and tear.

A work area that forces people to hold one shoulder
higher than another or causes them to bend the spine or neck
to one side can contribute to RSI.

A common problem for people working at computers is
their tendency to roll their shoulders forward, round their
lower backs, and thrust their chins forward. This posture becomes more pronounced when you're tired. Such posture
shortens the neck and shoulder muscles and lengthens the
upper back muscles, creating an imbalance. Muscles work best
at specific lengths. When they are unable to work at those
lengths, pain and tightness result. Eventually, the neck muscles
get tight and other muscles are substituted to do the task at
hand, and pain can develop in the neck, shoulders, and between the shoulder blades.

Such a posture may not even feel unbalanced because, as
creatures of habit, our bodies quickly conform to whatever
postures we adopt. The elasticity of ligaments and other connective tissues means that they tend to spring back to their
normal position. So gradually, you actually train your body to
conform to a particular posture.

Over time, bad posture can lead to chronic pain and discomfort and can be difficult to reverse.

Problem Postures

A number of specific postures can lead to RSI. You may be doing them and not even notice the discomfort either because it seems like such a small thing, or it has become habit. Moreover, if you are feeling pain, you may not feel it at the site of the awkward posture, but in another part of your body, which can be confusing. But posture is key, especially if you're already injured.

Here are some postures to avoid:

Cradling a telephone A common problem is cradling a phone receiver between your head and shoulder while talking. This causes the joints, ligaments, and muscles on one side of the neck to be stretched, while the joints, ligaments, and muscles on the other side are shortened and compressed. That can lead to a neckache, headache, and if done a great deal on one side, even a pinched nerve. Using a telephone headset can help a great deal. If you can't use a headset for some reason, switch sides regularly.

Arms unsupported and extended away from your body Sitting at a desk that is too high for you—another common problem in companies that simply put computer keyboards on desks previously used for typewriters or other equipment—forces you to lift your shoulders and hold your arms away from your body, which can cause shoulder and neck cramps.

Reaching for a computer mouse on a surface that is too high or too low forces you to reach out with your arm and can cause arm and shoulder pain. Gripping it tightly can lead to wrist pain.

Constantly reaching—overhead or behind your back, for example—for work materials from a constrained position has been linked to neck aches, shoulder tendinitis, and thoracic outlet syndrome. Supermarket cashiers have reported a range of RSIs, and some researchers believe that shoulder problems often found in cashiers are associated with sorting and moving merchandise past price scanners.

One shoulder higher than another   Women often joke about carrying around their lives in their purses. But carrying a heavy shoulder bag forces one shoulder to be higher than another. Photographers, who routinely carry heavy bags of equipment on their shoulders, and letter carriers, who carry mailbags, find themselves forced into the same awkward posture. Researchers have linked that posture to shoulder tendinitis and thoracic outlet syndrome.

Bending the wrist up and back   This is a particular problem with older, thicker computer keyboards that can force the user to cock the wrist up. Anytime the wrist is bent, more effort is required to complete a task than when the wrist is in a neutral position. Tenosynovitis of the forearm can result. Even though the wrist is being stressed, the muscles in the forearm are being overloaded as a result of that posture.

Bending the wrist sideways, toward the thumb   This can happen when trying to hit the space bar on some keyboards, or when twisting the lid of a jar. Done repeatedly, this irritates the tendon attachment of the finger extensor muscle that originates on the outside of the elbow. It can cause De Quervain's disease and/or tenosynovitis.

Bending the wrist toward the little finger   This is a particular problem on keyboards that have function keys off to the side or above the standard rows of keys. Once the wrist is out of a neutral position—like the standard handshake position—a proportional decrease in strength results. Constantly striking keys from that weak position can cause pain and soreness in the wrist and/or De Quervain's disease.

Holding the elbow straight while extending the arm   This posture is likely to cause shoulder problems. When the arm is extended, the flexor muscles can only produce weak lifting or pulling actions. Any task that requires more than a weak effort from that position may strain the arm.

Shoulders hunched forward or raised   This position can cause neck and shoulder strain. People commonly exhibit increased tension in the shoulder with typing, especially if the surface is high.

Pressing the back of the hand against a sharp edge   The backs and sides of fingers are sensitive to excessive pressure because the skin is thinner there. Using scissors over a long period of time can cause nerve problems in the fingers.

Resting the elbow or elbows on a hard surface   Leaning on a hard surface such as a desk or hard chair arms can cut off blood flow and eventually lead to compression of the nerves.

To some people, this all sounds a little silly. George, who is a writer's representative, jokes about his preferred typing posture: leaning far back in his chair, keyboard in his lap, and one leg thrown over another chair. When he worked for a large company, he says, he worried about the "ergonomics police" coming to get him. But RSI snared him as well, and he says he has learned that paying attention to posture pays off. (See Figure 3.1.)

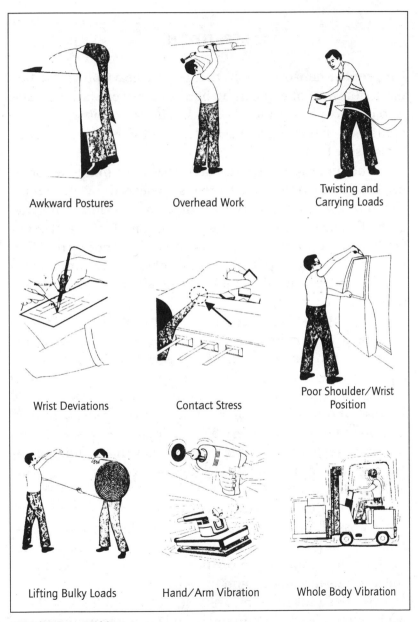

FIGURE 3.1: Problem postures

Reprinted from "Elements of Ergonomics Programs," National Institute of Occupational Safety and Health, 1997.

✂
REPETITION

For people who work in jobs that require heavy physical labor, the seriousness of RSI can be hard to believe. Maria, a nurse who lifts people day after day, asks, "How can a little repetitive motion do that much damage when I lift sick people and all I get is a sore back?"

The more repetitive the task, the more muscle effort is needed. At the same time, more rest is needed for those muscles to recover from the contractions. The fine-motor muscles of the fingers, hands, and arms are not built for tens of thousands of repetitions a day without corresponding rest. But with the use of computers in most jobs and at home, many people are doing just that: making tens of thousands of repetitions without any break.

With typewriters, people get scores of minibreaks from the repetitive exercise of typing—changing paper, correcting errors, or even fixing a jammed key. Now that computers have replaced typewriters, all those minibreaks have been eliminated. Achieving a high rate of speed on a typewriter required a typist who had been trained; but with computers, even an untrained typist can achieve a fairly high rate of speed. And computer keyboards are able to do so many more functions—moving around paragraphs, deleting sections, or transposing words—all at the touch of a few keys.

Add to that the even greater capabilities of computers made possible in recent years by technological advances—E-mail, print preview, and surfing the Web. Each new advance translates into more and more time at the computer keyboard and less time moving around the office.

All that adds up to more keystrokes—hundreds of thousands of them. David Thompson, Ph.D., professor emeritus of industrial engineering at Stanford University and an ergonomic consultant, points out how quickly the keystrokes can add up. If you type sixty words a minute for six hours a day, you will hit an average of 108,000 keystrokes a day. And the faster you type, the more keystrokes. Occupational researchers have positively linked the number of keystrokes to the severity of injury, but they are just beginning to figure out what a safe number of keystrokes is. One researcher believes that typing more than twelve thousand to fourteen thousand keystrokes an hour is dangerous. However, there may be no safe number of keystrokes because force, posture, workplace layout, and other factors play a role in causing RSI.

Besides, unless your work is electronically monitored, it's difficult to figure out how many keystrokes you do in a day. Most doctors treating RSI recommend limiting the time spent at a keyboard. The Japanese government has set a limit of three hundred minutes, or five hours, a day, which officials say has led to fewer RSIs among keyboard operators. However, current research indicates that limiting typing to even less time—four hours a day—may be safer because that appears to be the point at which the rate of injury rises. Job sharing has the same effect of limiting time at a keyboard.

Repetitive motion is not limited to working on a computer keyboard. Assembly-line work and playing music are other occupations where repetition is a physical hazard.

Researchers from the National Institute for Occupational Health Safety who studied telecommunications workers found that repetition and force were important factors in wrist and hand disorders reported by workers.

FORCE

It's probably surprising to know that even small tasks can place a load on muscles, adding up to hundreds of pounds of force. The more force required, the more muscle effort required. And the more muscle effort, the greater the decrease in the blood supply to the tissues and increased muscle fatigue.

In fact, fatigue is probably the most significant problem resulting from the force needed to complete a task. While researchers are still sorting out the complex measures of force and its implications, it is clear that muscle fatigue resulting from forceful movements can become chronic. Once certain muscles are fatigued and no longer able to handle the work load, other muscles that are not designed to do the particular task at hand take over. That leads to undue stress on those muscles.

When keyboarding, it is not uncommon for so-called experts to advise you not to pound the keys. That's difficult to do when you're in the middle of a project and concentrating on writing or calculating instead of the way your fingers are moving. One solution used by some is to put tiny pads, like those used for corns, on your keys as a way to provide cushioning.

It's more realistic, however, to expect equipment manufacturers to design keyboards to minimize the impact of force. Engineers who have studied the force required to press down a computer key recommend that keyboards have either tactile or auditory *feedback*. That means that when you strike a key, you should hear a click or feel a slight snap or release to pressure. (Auditory feedback, however, is less preferable because it can disturb others working nearby.)

It's a small design component that can make a big difference because it prevents you from striking the hard bottom of the keyboard with the same force. Without that feedback, you are more likely to exert the same force until you hit bottom, which sends a tiny physical shock that reverberates up through your fingers, hands, and arms. It would be like a jogger running a marathon barefoot: Soon, the constant impact would do serious damage to the jogger's knees. The same thing can happen to your hands. The fingertips are sensitive—blind people use them to read braille, Professor Thompson points out.

The force you exert on a keyboard may seem inconsequential, but it is, in fact, substantial, Thompson says. If you type at the rate of sixty words a minute for six hours a day, you are hitting 108,000 keystrokes. If each keystroke takes *one extra ounce*, that is an extra ten thousand ounces of force per day, which is more than six thousand pounds or three tons! The amount of force required to strike keys varies from keyboard to keyboard, and clearly, every ounce makes a difference.

Researchers also have found that the fingertip force you need to complete a task is increased when you work with diminished sensation in your hands, such as the kind caused by vibration, exposure to cold, or wearing gloves.

Poor posture and force are often intertwined. Having to perform a task that requires a great deal of force from an unstable posture can overload the muscles and cause problems.

✄
DURATION

The length of time you spend at a particular activity—in terms of hours and in terms of years—appears to be associated with injury. Study after study indicate that the rate of injury goes up the longer you do a particular activity without taking a break. A survey of the Music Teachers National Association, for example, found a highly significant relationship between the hours spent playing or teaching and the frequency of injuries.

In addition, it appears that more injuries in the workplace occur among employees who have been on the job for a while. That sometimes confuses people, who wonder why they didn't experience symptoms when they first started work. In fact, some do. Others only become aware of symptoms after a period of time. This injury is cumulative; that is, it occurs over time.

VIBRATION

Vibration causes constriction of the blood vessels and can lead to nerve damage. It has been linked to Raynaud's phenomenon. Symptoms of Raynaud's disease include intermittent numbness and tingling in the fingers, pale skin, feeling cold, and eventual loss of sensation and function in the hands.

People with RSI have reported that any activity involving vibration—riding in a train or plane or bicycling, for example, sparks their symptoms.

POOR WORKSTATION AND EQUIPMENT DESIGN

Most workstations and the equipment used with them are designed for the average body. Unfortunately, that body doesn't exist.

Even if you are of average height and weight you have different physical strengths, weaknesses, and habits from other people. Occupational engineers and ergonomists have a cardinal rule: Make the equipment fit the person, not the other way around.

In the workplace, however, it is generally the other way around. Almost an entire department of a large New York company was afflicted with RSI after a remodeling added more desks and computers to an already-crowded space. The new workstations were several inches shorter and narrower than the previous ones, and people complained of feeling crowded. Those few inches made a big difference, as worker after worker, forced into cramped positions by the new workstations, exhibited RSI.

Again, posture is intertwined with workstation and equipment design. Bad design can force you into a posture you might not even notice but that can be risky. (More on proper workstation and equipment design will be discussed in chapter 5.)

In general, equipment that is not adjustable can pose a problem. Common problems include a work surface that is too high or too low, a workstation that requires you to do unnecessary twisting or reaching, and equipment that does not provide adequate support for the arms. Crowding can also be a problem if it forces workers into a constrained posture.

Keyboards are a controversial topic because they are the subject of scores of lawsuits across the country. A growing number of researchers believes they can pose a problem as well. An extremely thick keyboard forces workers to cock up their wrist when typing, which can lead to compression of the median nerve. One lacking in feedback allows fingers to hit bottom without any cushioning effect. The poor placement of function keys can mean that you have to continually strike a frequently used key with a weaker finger, like the pinkie finger.

Some researchers believe that even a standard keyboard without design defects may pose problems. The flatness of the standard keypad forces you to arch your fingers, causing tension across the back of the hand. The rectangular shape of the keypad forces the hands to stay fairly close together, causing the forearms to rotate inward. In addition, the shape of the standard keypad encourages you to bend your wrist toward the pinkie to reach certain keys. Increasingly, keyboard manufacturers are experimenting with the design of keyboards in an effort to achieve a more comfortable unit.

Researchers are studying the differences among traditional and the so-called alternative keyboards. Alternative keyboards attempt to allow you to place your hands in a more neutral position while typing, which means that the muscles and tendons of the hands and arms are under little pressure because no awkward positions are assumed. To achieve a neutral posture, like the handshake position, designers have come up with split and vertically inclined keyboards.

Two 1997 keyboard studies—one by Marquette University and the other by the National Institute for Occupational Safety and Health—did not show that alternative keyboards prevent RSI. However, the Marquette study found that the alternative keyboards greatly reduced one important risk factor: wrist ulnar deviation, which is moving the wrist toward the little finger. The study, conducted over two days on people who had no symptoms of RSI, found no difference in discomfort levels between alternative and traditional keyboards but did find that the alternative keyboards positively affected posture. Given the significance of posture as a risk factor, that is a noteworthy finding, which, unfortunately, has been given short shrift in national coverage.

✄
JOB DESIGN

Changing your workstation so that it accommodates the body won't make much of a difference if you haven't paid attention to what occupational researchers call "work organization," or job design. They have found two key factors in job design that contribute to RSI: work load and the pace of work.

Work Load

Although the causes of RSI are still under investigation, evidence is fairly strong on one point: The longer and harder you work, the more likely you are to get injured. Here the issue of duration is key: If you take few or no breaks and work harder at the end of the day or the week—when your hands and arms are likely to be the most fatigued—you incur greater risk.

The National Institute of Occupational Safety and Health and the University of Michigan scientists who conducted a 1990 study of *Newsday*, a daily newspaper on Long Island, where hundreds of employees have reported symptoms of RSI, found that the hardest workers were the most severely injured. In general, employees who typed faster, spent longer periods of time typing, and took fewer breaks were more likely to be injured. That finding has been replicated in other studies.

The issue of work load poses a quandary for companies where downsizing has left remaining employees with more work. It is also an issue for laid-off workers who have taken temporary jobs at lower pay in the hopes of getting a permanent jobs. Many people have to work two jobs just to get by financially. Others, who know that doing a job well is no guarantee of job security, seek additional training in their off-hours. Workers in a variety of industries are shouldering a heavier work load.

To cope, some physicians advise patients to avoid working overtime, if possible. Or they suggest talking to a supervisor about getting extra help. That may be worth a try, but it probably won't get very far. Very likely, the manager is worried about her own job security and is unwilling or unable to change the work load.

If that's the case, it may be more practical to try to change the way you do your work. If possible, vary your duties. It can make the job more interesting and limit the amount of time you are engaged in an injurious activity, like typing. If you must work a second job, try to take one that involves a different kind of physical activity.

If RSI is associated with keyboarding, think of ways to cut down on typing. For example, rather than E-mailing, or messaging a coworker via computer, it makes sense to get up and talk to your coworker. Instead of taking notes on a computer, take them by hand. Or you can create macros to cut down on keystrokes. Varying your tasks may mean you work a little less efficiently, but it can help save your hands and arms. When dealing with RSI, small steps can certainly make a big difference.

Work load is a difficult issue because it also is wrapped up in your own sense of your professional identity. It may not be your boss pushing you to work long and hard; it may be your own professional pride driving you. Some people label hard workers as *driven*, or *obsessed*, but, in fact, our corporate culture encourages people to work hard. And there is nothing wrong with that—as long as it doesn't hurt you.

After Wendy, a public relations executive, came down with RSI, she confided to a friend that it was probably her fault because she worked so hard. Her friend, a little older and wiser, looked at her levelly and said, "That's *why* they hired you, because you work too hard."

So the matter of a work load that is too heavy may be a matter of negotiating not with a boss, but with yourself. It may be a matter of setting limits, if possible. Or it may necessitate changing to a job that allows greater flexibility. There are no easy answers.

But remember: It's your body, not the company's. *You* are the one who must live with the consequences of any injury.

Pace of Work

One of the big benefits that companies have heralded with the advances of technology is that it allows workers to do more work, faster. Experts love to cite statistics showing how much faster a computer can do a task than a human being can. And many managers love the fact that computers enable them to quantify workers' productivity in ways that were never possible before. The effect of these technological advances has been to increase the pace of work.

That being the case, it becomes critical to take breaks. Researchers have found that taking breaks of ten to fifteen minutes every few hours—as is standard in many workplaces—is not helpful in preventing RSI. It's far more helpful to take shorter, more frequent breaks. The longer you put off taking a break, the longer your body may be forced to remain in a constrained posture. When concentrating on a task, it's often tough to break away because you want to get it done. But there are ways to give your body much-needed minibreaks.

Many professionals treating RSI now advise patients to take a few minutes or even seconds to stretch every hour or so. One journalist, who was out of work for six months because of RSI and now is back at work full time, has made frequent stretches such a habit that he doesn't even think about them. Sometimes, he says, he'll find himself stretching at a party and getting funny looks from other guests.

It also makes sense to get up and walk around for a few moments. Even shifting position in your chair or at the desk can give your body a break. For people whose work is electronically monitored, those little breaks can be difficult to accomplish. If you have to raise your hand to go to the bathroom, as Eileen did in her data entry job at an insurance company, it's not likely you'll be able to get up and walk around much.

Electronic monitoring is common in the workplace. It's cheap and effective. Most, if not all, office computer systems have as a standard feature the capability to monitor an employee's work. That, of course, has raised concerns about privacy and the prospect of treating human beings as interchangeable parts. The more immediate concern for anyone dealing with RSI is how monitoring affects the pace of work.

The computer's ability to time and count keystrokes enables managers to set stringent quotas on time and productivity. High rates of stress, as well as muscle complaints have been found among clerical workers whose keystrokes are monitored, and airline reservations clerks whose statistics are frequently checked. A 1990 study of occupational stress conducted by the University of Wisconsin and the Communication Workers of America found a strong link between electronic monitoring and psychological and physical complaints. Workers who were monitored reported more boredom, tension, fatigue, and musculoskeletal problems than those whose work was not monitored.

Employers argue that they have a right to monitor work done on their equipment on their premises. Union activists counter that while short-term productivity may be boosted by monitoring, long-term productivity suffers because workers are so damaged by it. Some European countries regulate the use of electronic monitoring, but it remains unrestricted in the United States. The debate on the issue is unlikely to abate anytime soon.

✄

STRESS

Stress is a hot-button issue for some because it's often used to blame the victim. People suffering from stress are frequently advised to change the way they respond to the stressful situation rather than changing the situation itself. That addresses the symptoms, not the cause—and it doesn't always work. One occupational physician argues that stress-management courses usually target the wrong people because they're aimed at workers, not managers.

If you are experiencing symptoms of stress, there probably is a good reason for it. *It's your body's reasonable response to unreasonable demands.*

Stress causes a wide range of physiological changes in the body. Muscles under stress contract more and relax less, which results in a diminished blood flow and a buildup of metabolic wastes like lactic acid in the affected areas. There is also the well-known "fight or flight" response, whereby the body sends out hormones that provide the extra energy, alertness, and strength needed to complete a task. Yet another way the body responds to stress is to simply shut down.

Those physiological changes manifest themselves in a number of ways. Some physical signs of stress include:

- fatigue, loss of energy
- insomnia, inability to fall asleep and/or stay asleep
- eyestrain
- headaches, neck strain
- muscle strain, soreness
- irregular menstrual periods
- stomach problems

Because most people have so much going on in their lives at any one time, it's difficult to pinpoint what is merely temporary and what may be due to a long-term problem. Often, if the problem is ongoing, the physical signs of stress will be accompanied by psychological symptoms. Some of those include the following:

- irritability, anger
- inability to concentrate
- boredom, feeling dissatisfied, even when doing activities that previously brought pleasure

- feeling overwhelmed
- depression, a sense of powerlessness
- feeling unable to relax without drugs or alcohol

The causes of stress in the workplace range from the physical, for example, being forced to sit in an unstable or constrained posture for long periods of time, to the psychological, for example, working in a job where you have little control over the pacing or type of work you do. When dealing with stress, figure out its cause. This is sometimes hard to do. It's easy to blame a job for all your stress, but a job may not be the whole story. Be honest with yourself. If necessary, take some time off to evaluate your situation, or talk to someone about it. That way, you should be able to determine what you can change and what you cannot. You may not need to make a drastic change. You may be able to solve the problem by making a small change.

Researchers from the National Institute for Occupational Safety and Health who studied telecommunications workers in 1992 found that what they called *psychosocial factors*—fears about job security and lack of control over work—were related to neck and shoulder disorders. The institute has been doing further research on the physical effects of stress, including whether the release of the stress hormone cortisol reduces blood flow to contracted muscles. Another area of research is whether stress-prone workers tend to ignore symptoms—and as a result end up more severely injured.

It is impossible to eliminate stress from our lives; nor would we want to. Stress can be a positive experience, whether it's completing a tough job on deadline or running a race. It becomes dangerous if your body is forced to respond to stress over prolonged periods because that takes a physical and psychological toll. It's important to pay attention to your body before it reaches its breaking point.

The causes of RSI are complex and likely to be the source of debate for years to come. Your susceptibility to RSI is influenced by certain risk factors, some of which you can change. Reducing your risk could make the difference between mild or severe symptoms, a case that lasts only a short time or one that lasts much longer.

CHAPTER 4

WHO IS AT RISK FOR RSI?

✄

Lauren, the office manager for a small company in the Southeast, recalls her sense of shock when her doctor diagnosed the burning pain she had been feeling in her forearms for months as work-related tenosynovitis. Her doctor, an occupational physician, told her that her RSI was as bad as the cases he had seen among his patients who worked boning chicken all day long. "Who in the world would think you could get this badly hurt working in an office? It's not like I ever knew this was a high-risk job," she says.

✄
ANYONE IS AT RISK

Who's at risk for RSI? A wide range of occupations, especially workers who use a computer as a regular part of their job.

Just because you work at a computer does not mean you will develop RSI. And it is not limited to computer users. Workers in many other occupations have reported cases of RSI, in fact, in higher numbers than computer users. But the increasing dependence on computers, both at home and work, has helped cause the rates of RSI cases among computer users to skyrocket. It is important to be aware that typing at a computer is not as benign as it seems, as Lauren found out. The American Academy of Orthopedic Surgeons, which analyzed twenty of the largest studies of RSI among workers who use computers, found that spending just four hours a day at the keyboard increases your risk of shoulder, arm, wrist, and hand disorders two to three times that of someone who spends less time at the computer.

Assessing your own risk for RSI is fairly easy once you become aware of the problem. Researchers have identified a number of risk factors. Some you can change; others you can't. Changing what you can may be enough to mitigate the problem. This does not let manufacturers or employers off the hook when it comes to providing safe equipment and safe workplaces. But understanding the complex interactions of the body with a tool like a computer can help you take control of your health. Risk factors include:

- How hard you work
- How you work
- Heredity
- Gender
- General health
- Activities outside work

Following are some case studies of people who developed RSI. There is no common thread in these cases; they serve to illustrate that a variety of risk factors is at work in the development of RSI. Causation is complex. Looking at risk factors is valuable because it can help you eliminate or mitigate any factors that might contribute to the problem. Consider these cases:

> *One woman in her thirties worked not on one, but two, computer monitors in her job as a newspaper copy editor. She needed one terminal to read and edit copy and the other to handle the computerized page layout and design. At night she worked on a continual deadline because she edited several editions. The pressure was constant. It was not unusual for her to read more than thirty stories in a night. In addition, neither keyboard was easy to reach because she had to squeeze both onto one workstation. She felt burning pains in her forearms but worked through it until she couldn't do it any longer. Her arms simply gave out.*

> *A young man who worked in a meat-packing plant knew what could happen to his hands on the job. Everybody did. The plant was cold, like a refrigerator, and the pace unrelenting. He and his partner split one hundred and seventy-five carcasses an hour. The floor and tools were slippery from blood and grease. He occasionally cut himself. Sometimes, he'd see a guy trying to pry open his hands in the morning. Though he is a strong man, his grip is gone. He's already had two operations, and he's back at work and in pain.*

> *The violinist was a middle-aged man who loved to perform but hated rote warmups. He paid little attention to his posture while playing because he was so absorbed in the music. When a performance neared, he would spend hours perfecting the piece. By the time*

the performance was over, his hands would ache. In his time off, he would spend hours on his home computer, surfing the Internet. For a while, he ignored the aching in his hands. Then, one day, he found he couldn't hold the bow.

❧

HOW HARD DO YOU WORK

Though RSI sufferers often complain that coworkers secretly (or not so secretly) think they're malingering when they're injured, it is, in fact, the hardest workers who are hurt. Barbara Silverstein, an epidemiologist who has studied RSI extensively, told the *New York Times* in an interview, "It is the high-performance people who are at highest risk of musculoskeletal disorders." Physical therapists who worked with RSI patients confirm that same observation: It is the high achievers, the hard-driving workers who are hardest hit.

An intriguing study at a Ford Motor Co. Plant in Lansdale, Pennsylvania, monitored workers' muscle fatigue after particular tasks with electromyographs (EMGs), which measure muscle activity through electrical impulses. The study found that workers with RSI put twice as much effort into their jobs as workers who had no symptoms of RSI.

It may be your choice to work hard, or it may not. Unions in the United States see the current drive to increase production and eliminate downtime as strong contributors to workplace injuries such as RSI. Australian occupational studies of RSI found higher rates of RSI in companies with bonus and incentive plans tied to production; staff shortages forcing remaining workers to take on more work; and jobs requiring high amounts of overtime. The reason is simple: Under any of those conditions, workers are forced to work longer and harder when their bodies are tired and most vulnerable to injury.

Longtime employees are at risk: The length of time you've been working at a job can be a factor because RSI develops over a long period. It takes hundreds of thousands of keystrokes to cause injury, a number that can only be achieved over time.

Some of the most severely injured people are those who worked through their pain, either because they didn't understand what was happening to their bodies or they were so dedicated to their jobs—or both. In the hard-driving U.S. corporate culture, that's not uncommon. In fact, such dedication is often a source of pride among employees and managers alike.

Take the case of Carol, a key data operator with a state agency in California. She woke up one morning unable to open her left hand without prying the fingers apart with her other hand. She could not turn a doorknob or shampoo her hair, but went to work anyway and typed with her right hand.

A neurologist diagnosed her with carpal tunnel syndrome due to her work and predicted that she would develop similar symptoms in her right hand if she continued working, according to a report published by *9 to 5 National Association of Working Women*, in which Carol's case was described. The neurologist recommended that she change occupations, quit work, or go on welfare.

Carol clearly had pride in her work and had been a dedicated employee for fifteen years. She was not ready to quit. "I stick with it 'cause I'm fast, I'm efficient, I'm good. I go to work every day and earn my money and pay my bills. As long as I have one hand, I'll go on working."

Employers love Carol's can-do enthusiasm, but it's a high-risk activity, particularly for someone already experiencing symptoms.

In the case of Al, a well-respected fifty-five-year-old journalist in Minneapolis, it was a matter of his thinking that age
had caught up with him. When he first started noticing symptoms a few years ago, he says he thought, "Well, you know, I'm
starting to fall apart." He initially didn't think much of the
pain he was experiencing until one day he felt a "hot, running
pain" while doing some sanding work at home.

He was diagnosed with RSI. His employer has been extremely supportive, Al says, and has provided him with a
voice-activated computer so that he can continue to work. Although Al feels he has his RSI "well under control" and is
loathe to complain, he still must be careful about the way he
does simple chores, like carrying shopping bags. His symptoms were far more than "old" age causing him to fall apart.

In fact, it's not just longtime employees who develop RSI.
Alarmingly, cases have been reported among younger and
younger patients, from graduate students struggling to finish
theses to teenagers hooked on video games. (More on that will
be discussed later in this chapter.)

❧
HOW DO YOU WORK

Your style of working—both physical and mental—can influence your risk of developing RSI.

As mentioned in chapter 3, posture is key. If you use a
workstation that forces you into a constrained posture for
long periods of time, you could develop a problem.

One man, who has a business selling eyeglasses and contact lenses out of a storefront in a small shopping center, recently noticed sharp pains in his wrists and a nagging ache in
his neck. He started to worry when the pains didn't go away

on the weekends. A coworker urged him to get some advice on how to set up his computer, which he used much of the day. He had placed it on top of an eyeglass-display case, with the keyboard nearly a foot to the left of the monitor, which was set down well below his shoulders. And he sat on a stool without arm or back support. Advised to adjust his monitor and to buy a good chair and wrist rest, his pains went away. He still cannot believe that such seemingly small changes made such a big difference in how his hands and arms feel.

Working in an environment that is crowded, noisy, and has inadequate ventilation can also contribute to the physical risks. You may not even feel the stress, but it can be significant over time. Your muscles tense and your blood circulation slows down when you're under that kind of stress, setting you up for injury.

Pace of work is important as well. If you work on a computer system that experiences frequent system breakdowns, you could be forced to speed up and complete a task in less than the optimal time. Being unable to control when you take breaks or being unable to take frequent breaks overloads muscles and tendons. Studies have consistently linked a lack of control over pace of work with RSI.

Doing the same task again and again puts muscles and tendons at risk because of the repetition. Occupational physicians recommend varying work tasks whenever possible.

Working on deadline or having to handle sudden increases in work load are contributing risk factors because you are forced to work when you are most tired, or to work through pain—both of which can damage muscles and tendons. Muscles need time to relax. Stress can increase muscle tension, which leads to increased muscle fatigue and pain, setting up a vicious cycle.

A number of occupations have reported significant rates

of RSI. They include the jobs and corresponding risky activities shown in Table 4.1.

This list is by no means complete. It is intended to give you a sense of how widespread the problem of RSI is. Though nonwork-related factors may contribute to RSI, as will be discussed below, working conditions are clearly significant

HEREDITY

Each of us has different inherited strengths and weaknesses. That helps to explain why when two people do the same job—say, type at a computer keyboard—one may be severely debilitated by RSI and the other is not affected at all. It is not uncommon for someone afflicted with RSI to be asked—often in a disbelieving tone—by a healthy coworker: "We do the same job. Why did you get it and not me?"

That's like asking why one person on the block got cancer and his next-door neighbor did not.

Each of us carries in our bodies a different set of predispositions. In fact, recent research, in which study subjects were asked to detail their family histories, indicates that there may be an inherited predisposition to carpal tunnel syndrome. The physiological mechanisms that may be involved are not clear. In addition, tensile tendon strength and resistance to injury can vary from individual to individual.

One physical trait that has been linked with RSI is double-jointedness. Some researchers believe that double-jointedness means that the hands and wrists bounce more in repetitive activities, causing even more dangerous repetitions. Beyond that, however, the research on just what else may predispose a person to RSI is fairly limited.

TABLE 4.1: OCCUPATIONS AT RISK

Occupation	Risks
Assembly-line workers	Repetition, reaching overhead or twisting to the side, thumb pressure, pinch grip, ulnar deviation, little control over pace of work.
Pieceworkers	Hunching shoulders, flexing wrists.
Meat cutters	Twisting hands, extending and flexing wrists with force, little control over pace of work.
Typists, data entry operators	Static posture, repetition, bending wrists.
Journalists	Static posture, deadline work, bending wrists.
Telephone operators	Bending wrists, prolonged posture that puts pressure on elbows, little control over pace of work.
Airline reservationists	Repetition, little control over pace of work, static postures.
Musicians	Repetition, hunching shoulders, forceful wrist motions.
Graphic designers	Gripping with fingers, hunching shoulders.
Supermarket cashiers	Pulling, lifting and twisting wrists, repetition.
Construction workers	Repetition, awkward postures, use of vibrating tools.
Postal workers	Repetition, flexing wrists, pressure on shoulder from carrying a mailbag.
Glass cutters	Prolonged posture that puts pressure on bent elbows.
Flight attendants	Flexing wrists, pushing heavy food carts.
Welders	Static postures, vibration.
Electricians	Twisting wrists forcefully.

The issue of inherited risk factors is a touchy one because some unions fear employers will call for screening job applicants for these factors. Some employers argue that screening is not unreasonable because many companies already screen job applicants through physical exams and tests for illegal drug use. Unions argue that the work environment and job design are far more important risk factors, and that they should be addressed before any employee screening is done. It's unlikely that any extensive screening of this type will be done soon in the United States because there just isn't compelling evidence that inherited risk factors are more significant than others.

❃
GENDER

Roughly two out of three cases of RSI are women. While there are no consistent scientific findings to prove their theory, clinicians believe this is due to several factors. Women have generally smaller bone mass and muscles and thus are less able to absorb the impact of repeated insults to the body. Women also experience profound hormonal changes during pregnancy and menstruation, which can lead to swelling that, in turn, puts pressure on the tissues, causing a condition like carpal tunnel syndrome. Oral contraceptives, which mimic pregnancy, can also cause swelling.

The higher rates of RSI among women may be due to the fact that more women work in high-risk jobs. They also may be less likely to complain about working conditions out of fear of losing their jobs.

Although more women have RSI, statistics indicate that more men actually lose time from work as a result.

❊
GENERAL HEALTH

Your overall health can be a contributing risk factor—as it would be in any chronic illness or injury. In discussing these factors, it should be noted that they are not the cause of RSI but may well contribute to the severity of the injury. Doctors who try to blame a patient's RSI on smoking or obesity alone are simply ignoring or are ignorant of other documented risk factors, such as pace of work and badly designed equipment. The factors that are discussed here are included only to help you understand and minimize your own risk. Areas of concern include the following:

- An underlying physical condition such as diabetes or rheumatoid arthritis
- Fatigue
- An earlier trauma to the body
- Obesity
- Smoking
- Excessive alcohol use

A number of underlying physical conditions has been linked to RSI. Carpal tunnel syndrome has been diagnosed in people who have conditions that cause excess fluid retention, including diabetes, hypothyroidism, pregnancy, and some allergic reactions. Diabetes actually makes the nerves more sensitive to pressure. Rheumatoid arthritis, high blood pressure, and Lyme disease also have been implicated as contributors to RSI.

In some cases, these conditions are considered the primary cause of RSI. Pregnancy, for example, is considered a cause of carpal tunnel syndrome because it frequently causes swelling. However, it is not considered to be a cause of other

RSIs, like tenosynovitis, and, in fact, there have been anecdotal reports of some RSI patients (who do not have carpal tunnel syndrome) saying they feel better during pregnancy. That may be attributable to the hormonal changes and muscle laxity that occur during pregnancy.

There is some debate over whether diabetes is a cause of RSI. Some physicians believe it is, while others argue that diabetes creates an "eggshell" effect, in which the tissues are more prone to injury, and therefore the disease is only a contributing factor. Rheumatoid arthritis is considered a primary cause of RSI. The distinction between whether a condition is regarded as the primary cause or merely a contributing factor is not always clear-cut. It must be taken in consideration with other aspects of a patient's medical history.

Fatigue is important because tired muscles and tendons are more vulnerable to injury. It may be a matter of not getting enough sleep—a problem for many—or it may be a matter of doing too much work when arms are tired. A work load that increases toward the end of the day or the end of the week can force you to work hardest when your body is in need of rest. Like any machine, body parts wear out when they're overused or pushed beyond reasonable limits.

An earlier trauma to the body—for example, a broken bone or ligament tear due to a car accident or sports injury—might lead to problems because healthy muscles tend to compensate for weakened muscles. This may cause a postural imbalance in the body. One administrator from Long Island, New York, developed carpal tunnel syndrome after a car accident and found herself unable to do her job, which involved extensive typing on a computer.

Some prominent researchers believe obesity is a significant risk factor for RSI, in part because of the extra pressure excess weight puts on muscles and tendons. It also may be that overweight people are more likely to be forced into awkward postures by using a workstation and equipment designed for a smaller person. This is another touchy subject because of societal prejudice against overweight people. It is *not* the excess weight that causes RSI, but excess weight can make it worse.

Smoking is considered by some to be a risk factor because nicotine hampers blood circulation, which is essential to removing metabolic wastes that build up in muscles during high activity. However, since many workplaces force smokers to smoke in separate areas or outside the building, smoking actually may encourage people to take those much-needed breaks!

Occasional alcohol use is not considered a problem, but excessive alcohol use is. Alcohol is essentially a central nervous system depressant. It interrupts deep sleep, which contributes to fatigue. It also causes dehydration, which forces the body to work harder to do basic functions, such as circulation. And, in general, studies have shown that people who abuse alcohol tend to have other health problems, which may well contribute to RSI.

Alcoholics are susceptible to developing neuropathies that mimic carpal tunnel syndrome. They also can develop problems in proprioception, which is your three-dimensional sense of your body in your surroundings; this can contribute to RSI. Vitamin deficiencies are commonly seen among alcoholics because they tend to have poor nutritional habits, and some studies have linked a certain deficiency in vitamin B_6 to carpal tunnel syndrome, although that is still the subject of scientific debate. (B_6 and carpal tunnel syndrome will be discussed in more detail in chapter 9.)

ACTIVITIES OUTSIDE WORK

Hobbies that cause you to do repetitive or forceful motion and/or place you in an awkward posture can be a problem. Examples include playing video games, sewing, and carpentry.

RSI sufferers often ruefully complain of flareups after "doing something stupid" like painting a room or carrying heavy bags home from the grocery store. One woman carried luggage through several airports on a long-planned trip to Europe. She knew the exertion would set off her symptoms, but she could not bear the thought of canceling her trip.

Remember, you are perfectly entitled to use your arms doing chores around the house and in activities you enjoy—you used them for doing those things without even thinking about it before RSI. But it's worthwhile to note what activities may cause flareups so that you can do them carefully. Sometimes it's hard to pinpoint the activity causing you pain because you may not feel it until hours later; but over time, as you understand your body better, the pattern becomes more apparent.

Many RSI cases have been reported by musicians—professionals and amateurs. Pain and injury have been linked to long and intense practice sessions, cramped space, or poor placement of the chair or music stand. The location of pain tends to be specific to the instrument played; pianists, for example, tend to have pains in their right hands and arms; string players are more likely to be affected in the left hand. Physical therapists emphasize the importance of technique and posture in prevention of all types of RSI among musicians.

Many people with RSI complain that their symptoms flare up while driving. Holding your hands in the classic "10 and 2" position taught in driving schools can force you to hunch your shoulders and neck. It also forces you to bend your wrists, a highly uncomfortable position for people with carpal tunnel syndrome. A stick shift causes you to frequently flex and bend your wrists. Gripping a steering wheel tightly can put undue pressure on hands and fingers. Even merely riding in a car can set off symptoms for some because of the vibration and because being forced to hold a particular posture for any length of time forces muscles to contract.

Doing a second job or free-lance work that is similar to your primary job is risky because it puts additional strain on an already-overloaded set of muscles and tendons. The greater amount of time you spend doing an injurious activity, the greater the likelihood is that you will be injured.

✂

WHAT IS THE RISK AMONG YOUNG PEOPLE?

RSI develops over time, whether you feel it coming on or not. Until recently, most cases of RSI were reported among experienced workers who had been on the job for a number of years. That makes sense because young tendons are supple and resilient; as you get older, they become less resilient. However, as computers are used more widely in the home and schools, more and more cases have been reported among younger people. Federal statistics show increases among younger people, ages fourteen to twenty-five, who are sustaining work-related RSIs.

In fact, more and more people are sounding the alarm about the risk to young people. They point out that while many schools teach computer skills, they may not always teach proper keyboard placement or warn students of the risk of spending too much time at the computer.

At Harvard University, a group of graduate students formed an RSI support group. One computer-science student said in an interview with the *New York Times* that he had been unable to type for a year because of the severe pain of his RSI. "Everyone uses computers," he said. "And many more people are spending more time on computers. Before, if you wanted to talk to your friend, you had to get up and use the phone, or if you wanted to print something, you'd have to stop and print it out to see what it looked like. Now, you can do everything with e-mail, print preview, and the Web. You can sit there all day."

At the Massachusetts Institute of Technology, university officials have implemented a series of programs to make students more aware of the risk of developing a case of RSI. And a committee has been formed among school administrators to discuss ways to prevent injuries and help students who develop RSI.

RSI isn't limited to college students. A teenager sued the maker of the Nintendo video game because she had developed an RSI—what one rheumatologist called "Nintendinitis"—from playing the video game. The seventeen-year-old girl said her hands began tingling and went numb seven months after she started playing Nintendo several hours a day. She was diagnosed with carpal tunnel syndrome and found that her symptoms eased after she stopped playing. At the time, her lawyer said, "Welcome to Toyland." The case was settled, and the parties are barred from discussing the case further.

Of course, playing video games isn't limited to teenagers. It never occurred to one New Jersey man who worked on a computer in his job and developed severe RSI that his habit of playing video games all weekend might have contributed to his problem. He is not alone. People often fail to associate playing video games with overuse injuries, even though the physical activity of playing video games is similar to other kinds of computer-keyboard work.

The American Academy of Pediatrics reports no current research on the musculoskeletal effects of playing video games. The best advice for parents concerned about video games is to make sure their child is in a comfortable posture and to allow it only for limited amounts of time. It is when young people play for hours on end for months and years at a time that an overuse injury puts them at risk.

WHAT IS YOUR RISK OF CHRONIC INJURY?

RSI is frightening because it can be debilitating. The difference between being able to manage an injury or being disabled and unable to work is significant.

The risk of developing a chronic—and potentially disabling injury—is high if you choose to ignore the pain or try to "gut it out." Eventually, you'll reach a point where you'll simply be unable to ignore it.

Though it is never advisable to self-diagnose, understanding the severity of your RSI can help you assess your own risk of developing a chronic injury. No one should panic, but you should take it seriously—even if other people don't. Doctors have developed a variety of scales to measure the severity of RSI. Table 4.2 is one used by some physicians in Australia, where there was an outbreak of RSI in the early 1980s.

Checklist

To summarize, you can ask a number of questions when trying to assess your risk for RSI. Here is a brief checklist:

- If you keyboard, do you type more than three to four hours a day?
- Do you use your mouse more than six hours a week?
- Has your workstation been set up with ergonomic considerations in mind?
- Is work you do with your upper arms performed in an unsupported position away from the body?

TABLE 4.2: DEGREES OF INJURY

Degree of Injury	Characteristics of Pain	Remedy
Grade one	Pain is present only when performing the aggravating tasks; outside activities of daily living are not affected.	Modifications to workstation usually eliminate symptoms.
Grade two	Pain continues even after having stopped aggravating tasks; activities of daily living are affected to a small degree.	Modifications to workstation usually eases or eliminates symptoms.
Grade three	Pain continues long after work; activities of daily living are affected. Physical signs, such as tenderness or swelling, are present.	Patients at this level need rest. They usually can resume work after allowing themselves time to heal and if their workstations have been modified.
Grade four	Pain is present in the morning and usually at night, but may subside on weekends; activities of daily living are greatly affected.	Patients usually require lengthy time away from work. Recovery is uncertain, though not impossible.
Grade five	Pain is continuous; activities of daily living are substantially restricted.	Patients need lengthy period of time away from work. Recovery is uncertain.

- Are you able to take short, frequent breaks?
- Do you have control over the pacing of your work?
- Is your workplace noisy?
- Is your workplace excessively hot or cold?

- Are your work tasks varied?
- Are you a touch typist?
- Has there been a recent change in your job, like a change in workstation or increase in work load?
- Do you work on deadline?
- Are there enough people to do the job at your workplace?
- Are bonus or incentive plans tied to your production?
- Do you work a lot of overtime?
- Have you been on the job for long?
- Do you take oral contraceptives?
- Are you pregnant?
- Do you get enough sleep?
- Do you smoke?
- Do you drink excessive amounts of alcohol?
- Are you overweight?

There is no specific number of risk factors that should cause concern. Just how important a particular risk is depends on other aspects of your health. But if you answered "yes" to any of these questions, it is worthwhile to mention it to your doctor so that he can more accurately determine how best to treat you. There is no need to panic or jump to conclusions. These are merely risk factors, not indications of a problem. They are guidelines intended to help you understand how RSIs happen. Most risks can be eliminated or minimized. If you are concerned about a particular risk factor, talk to your doctor about it. You may be able to come up with an easy way to change it so that it no longer poses a risk.

CHAPTER 5

HOW TO PREVENT RSI

Betsy, a free-lance writer in New York, found herself unable to work for several months because of painful tenosynovitis, carpal tunnel syndrome, and cubital tunnel syndrome. While out of work, she underwent regular physical therapy, which she had to pay for on her own because she didn't have workers compensation insurance.

Betsy now has her symptoms under control but has had to change her pace of work and the kinds of projects she undertakes. She also has modified her work space in her apartment so that it meets ergonomic guidelines. Rather than spending a lot of money on specially designed ergonomic equipment, she has improvised many of the adaptations she needs. She has wrapped the edge of her desk with packing paper to soften the hard edge; uses a headset; relies on an elevated clipboard; and wraps moleskin around her pen so that she can write comfortably. To Betsy, improvising the ergonomic adaptations is "the fun part."

Although she can laugh about things like the funny-looking moleskin on her pen, Betsy is still mindful of the insidious nature of RSI and the risk people take if they don't think about ergonomics.

"I get furious when I read about the wonders of the computer, the Internet, and the World Wide Web, and the articles never, ever mention anything about the fact that the computer also presents dangers to its user," she says. "Everybody who uses the computer should make sure the equipment is ergonomically the best it can be. You need to remember that this is an instrument that can cause injury, and you need to protect yourself."

✂

REDUCING THE RISK OF GETTING HURT

Betsy's experience illustrates the fact that you *can* minimize your chances of getting hurt. It requires paying attention to "ergonomic" considerations, using well-designed equipment, and working in a sensible way.

Simply put, the term "ergonomic" means adapting the work environment to the human body. A multidisciplinary specialty area, it involves knowledge of human anatomy; biomechanics, or how muscular and skeletal systems operate during both static and dynamic work; the psychology of how people recognize and respond to signals; and industrial engineering, which is the design of workplaces and jobs themselves.

Ergonomics is a relatively new academic discipline, so new that some courts of law don't recognize it as a science. Nonetheless, many serious ergonomists have done and are doing important research on RSI that has already influenced the design of office equipment and some manufacturing plants. In the last decade, the demand for ergonomic equipment and advice has been so great that it has exploded into big business. And as with any new area where there is money to be made, more than a few so-called experts have popped up to sell a variety of products with questionable claims. It's easy to be fooled when something is simply labeled "ergonomic."

No one design fits everyone; so technically, an off-the-shelf product should not be labeled ergonomic unless it is completely adjustable. To protect yourself, it's important to understand the basic principles of ergonomics. But, remember, each person has different physical requirements, so if possible, consult someone with knowledge and experience in the field.

Although RSIs occur in a wide range of work environments, this chapter will detail setting up an ergonomic computer workstation because it's not feasible to discuss specific changes for every occupation, and computers are rapidly becoming ubiquitous at work and home. But the basic principles of paying attention to posture, choosing, and placing equipment so that it allows you to work comfortably apply to all kinds of jobs.

❈
CONSIDER POSTURE

Posture has been mentioned so much in this book that it's likely you're saying, "Not again!" But it needs to be discussed here because achieving a natural, balanced posture is one of the primary aims of ergonomic design. And that is important because it can help prevent injury.

The natural curvature of the spine, called lordosis, is shaped something like a sea horse, with the upper curve supporting the head and the lower curve supporting the upper body. A rigid, upright posture—the stereotypical notion of "good" posture—really isn't good. It forces the pelvis to rotate backward and straightens out the natural curve of the spine. In fact, a little slumping may not be bad. Forward slumping actually relaxes the large muscles that have to be tensed to hold us upright. That can ease pressure on the back.

In short, muscle activity is at a minimum when maintaining ideal posture, which translates into less wear and tear on the muscles. In addition, good posture minimizes the compressive forces on the disks of the spine, which, again, means less wear and tear on the spine.

When it comes to sitting at a workstation, the basic posture consists of the following: (See Figure 5.1.)

- The back should be angled slightly backward. That widens the angle between the torso and thighs, which should be greater than ninety degrees, increasing blood flow and reducing compression of the spine.
- Arms should be parallel to the floor, or angled slightly downward. It's helpful for some to have forearms supported by a wrist rest to relax the biceps and neutralize the wrist position.
- The thigh-torso angle should be greater than ninety degrees, and the knees should be at right angles to the thighs.
- Feet should be flat on the floor or on a comfortable footrest.
- The head should be balanced comfortably, the way you would hold it when you walk down the street.
- Wrists should be "neutral," that is, not cocked up or bent down.

Posture is difficult to change. Some people swear by the Feldenkrais or the Alexander Technique, which are systems of body work aimed at improving your natural posture. (This is discussed in chapter 10.) A more immediate solution is to

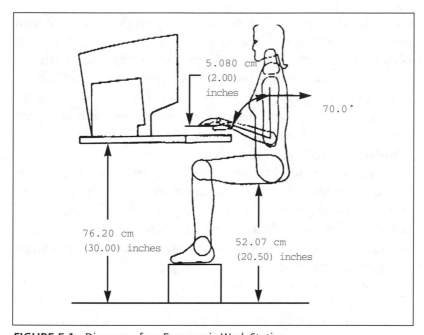

FIGURE 5.1: Diagram of an Ergonomic Work Station.

Reprinted with permisssion from American National Standard for Human Factors Engineering of VDT Workstations (ANSI/HFS 100-1988), 1988. Copyright by the Human Factors and Ergonomics Society.

modify the workstation so that you don't have to *think* about your posture.

❊
SETTING UP AN ERGONOMIC WORKSTATION

Companies that have made ergonomic changes to work areas have seen significant, and sometimes dramatic, drops in rates of RSI. Changes may be simple and inexpensive, like providing document holders and wrist rests to computer-keyboard users, or more elaborate and expensive, like redesigning an entire plant to place work surfaces at appropriate heights and place tools within easy reach. If you run your own business, it's incumbent on you to set up your work area with ergonomic considerations in mind. An ergonomic workstation not only can help prevent injury, it can help you continue to produce even after you are injured. Some people report that their symptoms have disappeared completely after they made adjustments to their workstation.

Given the potential expense, you may be tempted to skimp, especially if you're running your own business. However, it probably won't be necessary to spend thousands of dollars to get the right equipment. Many reasonably priced, well-designed ergonomic products are available. The equipment should be tried out before you purchase it. Most companies will let you try demonstration models for up to thirty days and then allow you to return the product if you don't like it. That way, you'll have a much better sense of what works for you. In addition, all business equipment and supplies you buy—desk, chairs, computers, and accessories—can be written off in the year they're purchased or can be depreciated over five- to seven-year periods.

The recommendations that follow are general guidelines; what's best for you may vary according to individual needs. "Remember, there is no average Joe or Jane," says Michael Gauf, managing editor of the *CTD News*, a monthly publication on current issues related to RSI. "Adjustability is one of the key factors when buying equipment."

Your Chair

Talk to any ergonomic consultant, and he will talk at length about the importance of chairs. In fact, some say it's the most important piece of office equipment you can buy. A virtual science of chairs has evolved as a result of all the research that's been done on chairs. There's even a fair amount of debate going on in the industry about whether a chair should be viewed as furniture—something you can use without thinking much about it, or as a tool—equipped with so many adjustable parts that you need an operator's manual to figure out how to use it.

And yet, in most offices, chairs are far more important as status symbols than as aids to your health. One woman who developed debilitating RSI after working in a production plant in Minneapolis remembers ruefully how difficult it was for her to get a chair with proper back and arm support at work because those chairs were reserved for managers, not administrative personnel.

But that attitude is changing. Canny observers of the O.J. Simpson criminal trial, noteworthy in part for how long it lasted, noticed that defense lawyers brought expensive, ergonomically designed chairs into the courtroom for themselves. Clearly, they knew they'd be in that courtroom for many hours, and they made sure they were in comfortable, well-designed chairs that they could adjust to their own bodies.

In selecting the right chair, two factors are key: support and adjustability. (See Figure 5.2.)

Though an entire chapter could be written about chairs alone (indeed, some people have written entire books about them), there are some specific design elements to consider when looking for a chair.

The back of the chair should allow you to recline and should provide support of some sort for the lower back. That support may range from a pillow that can be strapped onto the back to an air cushion built into the chair. A high back is helpful in providing upper-back support. A headrest isn't always necessary, but it can be important for someone who is experiencing neck and/or shoulder pain.

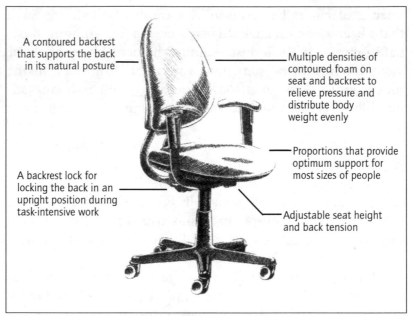

A contoured backrest
that supports the back
in its natural posture

Multiple densities of
contoured foam on
seat and backrest to
relieve pressure and
distribute body
weight evenly

Proportions that provide
optimum support for
most sizes of people

A backrest lock for
locking the back in an
upright position during
task-intensive work

Adjustable seat height
and back tension

FIGURE 5.2: Ergonomically Designed Chair.
As a rule of thumb, the more time you spend sitting at work and the more you
perform repetitive tasks, the more adjustability you need.
Reprinted with permission of Steelcase, Inc.

Armrests are the subject of some debate. Some people swear by them, others say they force them to hunch their shoulders. (Some chairs have armrests that are adjustable, both upward and downward, which eliminates that problem.) If you decide you need them, they should be padded and adjustable—up, down, in and out, if possible. If padding is not available, you can provide your own simply with foam rubber or bubble paper. It's not pretty, but it does the job.

The length of the seat pan should be from 13 to 19 inches, though that can vary, depending on your height. When you sit in the chair, there should be about 2 to 3 inches of space between the back of the knee and the point where the thigh hits the edge of the chair. The seat pan also should incline slightly forward and curve downward on the front edge. That helps maintain the natural curve of the spine and transfers pressure from the spine to the thighs and feet.

The height of the chair should allow you to place your feet flat on the floor. If that's not possible to do with your existing chair, you can buy a footrest or use a phone book.

The base of the chair should have five casters at the feet so that it is both sturdy and easily mobile.

A good chair does not have to be expensive. Good models are available for $300–$400. More expensive models, costing up to $2,400, are available, but it's not necessary for most people to spend that much money. Some vendors will offer a discount if you buy in volume. Buyers can cut the cost by choosing a medium-grade fabric rather than the most-expensive grade. (Besides, an expensive covering like leather actually isn't the best choice because it can increase the amount of slumping and sliding you'll do in the chair.) Most ergonomic experts will say that a good chair is worth the investment; and if it's used for business, it's tax-deductible. Consider the fact that a seat in a car costs in the range of $2,000; yet most people spend only about $100 on an office chair—where they are likely to spend far more time sitting.

To sum up, here's a quick checklist for a chair.

Chair Checklist

1. Is the chair easily adjustable from a seated position?
2. Can you adjust the backrest or easily modify it to provide lower-back support?
3. Does the back of the chair recline?
4. When you sit in the chair, are there about 2 to 3 inches of space between the back of the knee and the point where your thigh hits the edge of the chair?

5. Does the chair have a five-caster base?
6. When you sit in the chair, can you place your feet flat on the floor?

Your Desk

Like chairs, desks or work surfaces should be adjustable. In many offices, that's not the case. Again, it's often been more an issue of status than of practicality. But when computers are thrown on top of desks with no thought to appropriate heights or reach distances, problems can result. If, for example, you are tall and have gone to the trouble of getting an adjustable chair, you'll be cramped if you don't have adequate space under the desk. Or, if you are short or even of average height, most desks are set at a height that is comfortable for writing, not keyboarding.

Adjustable desks and work surfaces are available from furniture-supply stores in a range of models, from motorized to hand-cranked. Or, if you have a desk that you would rather modify, conversion kits are available to make it adjustable. An even simpler solution is to buy a computer table and place it next to the desk so that they form an L shape. That provides a comfortable height for writing and one for typing. If buying a new desk is not an option, you could buy an adjustable mount on which to place your keyboard.

Specific height recommendations vary. The American National Standards Institute recommends an under-desk leg clearance of 20.2 to 26.2 inches. A tall person may need more clearance.

For tasks other than keyboarding, a general rule of thumb offered by the National Institute of Occupational Safety and Health scientist Dr. Verne Putz Anderson in his book, *Cumulative Trauma Disorders*, is this: The more precise the work, the higher the work surface; the heavier the work, the lower the work surface.

It's important to organize a desk so that the most frequently used items are within easy reach. According to ergonomists, a well-organized work area should permit several different working positions, eliminating dangerous static loading on the muscles.

The tabletop should be thin to allow for sufficient legroom when typing. If you already have RSI, with acute symptoms, you may need to place padding on top of your work surface to prevent your arms and hands from coming into prolonged contact with sharp edges. Or, a wrist support could be used to protect your hands and arms.

Desk Checklist

1. Is your desk or work surface adjustable? If not, is there a way to make the area where you've placed a keyboard and monitor adjustable?
2. Is there enough room for your legs to fit comfortably and move around under the desk?
3. Is there enough space on your desk or work surface for the tools you need to do your job comfortably?

Your Keyboard and Monitor

Pages and pages could be written about the specifications for keyboards and monitors. A great deal of research is being done on both. In general, the basic thing to keep in mind while typing is to place a monitor so that the top of the screen is at eye level and below and to place the keyboard so that arms are parallel to the ground, or angled slightly downward, while typing. This way, the eyes are angled at approximately twenty degrees downward to read material. If you cannot place the keyboard so that your arms are parallel to the ground, it is preferable to have your arms angle downward rather than upward. It places far more strain on the arms if they're angled upward. That position puts more traction on the ulnar nerve, which runs through the "funny bone" in the elbow, by angling the elbows upward.

To achieve this posture, you should be able to detach the monitor from the keyboard. Most computer equipment—except laptops—is detachable. Laptops pose special problems because they're not adjustable. (Finding a way to work safely and comfortably on laptops will be discussed at the end of this section.)

To avoid angling your arms upward or cocking up wrists, the keyboard should be thin, with the home row set of keys (ASDFGHJKL) no higher than 1.25 inches from the base. That means that the home row should be at about elbow height.

To save your arms and hands from the hundreds of thousands of minishocks that come from the repetitive action of keying, ergonomists strongly recommend that your keyboard have audio or tactile feedback. That means that when the key is struck, there should be a noticeable click or slight spring that signals the finger to halt its downward motion before it hits bottom. You may not even be aware of it while typing, but it is critical. When a keyboard lacks that breakaway function, it means that your fingertips are bottoming out literally tens of thousands of times a day. If you consider that the typical full-time user of a computer keyboard makes one hundred thousand to a hundred and fifty thousand keystrokes a day, that is a lot of minishocks to absorb. Some occupational physicians recommend placing a pad of some sort under the keyboard to help absorb the shock as well.

The keys themselves should have a matte finish in order to cut down on glare and should be slightly concave, not flat, to accommodate the fingertips comfortably. Some physical therapists tell patients who are touch typists to put small pads, like corn pads, on each key to make them more comfortable.

Another factor to consider is the layout of the keyboard itself. Although the QWERTY layout is standard, the number and placement of function keys is not. Some keyboards have a large number of function keys, which is appealing to some users because of the variety of things they allow you to do. But researchers have found that hard-to-reach function keys that must be hit by weaker fingers, like the little finger of your weaker hand, can pose a danger. The more you have to strike a hard-to-reach key with your pinkie, the more likely it is that you will be injured. So in looking at the keyboard, the keys used should be those placed in easy-to-reach spots.

To avoid hunching the shoulders the recommended position for the monitor is to have the top of the screen placed at eye level or below. However, that may not be the best position for someone wearing bifocals. It is possible to get VDT glasses ground for VDT reading distance, but the simpler solution might be to place the monitor slightly lower than the recommended position. If you are nearsighted, it is often possible to go without glasses while typing. It may take some experimenting to find what's most comfortable. As far as viewing distance from the monitor, the National Institute of Occupational Safety and Health recommends keeping it 18 to 20 inches. You should place copy about as far away from your eyes as the monitor is so that your eyes don't have to refocus when shifting from the copy to the monitor.

The other big consideration with monitors is glare. Much headway has been made in recent years to reduce glare on the screen. In addition, good office designers often take it into consideration and recommend such things as indirect lighting to minimize glare. If you find glare to be a problem, you can probably reduce it by simply angling or tilting the monitor. If that doesn't work, a glare screen can be placed over the monitor. If you are sitting directly under overhead lights, a short hood over the terminal will reduce glare. If you can't find a hood, you can make one by taping black cardboard or construction paper around the top and sides of the monitor. When positioning a monitor, consider window placement. You are most likely to cut down on glare from sunlight by positioning your monitor perpendicular to windows and not directly facing them or away from them.

Keyboard and Monitor Checklist

1. Can the keyboard be detached from the monitor so that you can adjust it?
2. Is the keyboard thin and angled only slightly upward?
3. When you strike the keys, do you feel or hear a spring or feel the pressure slightly decrease so that you don't hit the keys too hard?
4. Can you shift and reach function keys without awkward straining?
5. Is your monitor placed at eye level or slightly below?
6. Is your monitor positioned to cut down glare?
7. Does your setup allow you to work with arms parallel to the floor and wrists straight?

Alternative Keyboards

If you are about to buy a keyboard, or need to change your equipment because you're suffering from RSI, it may be worthwhile to consider an alternative, or ergonomic, keyboard. Dozens of companies, prompted both by the explosion in the PC market and the scores of lawsuits filed against keyboard manufacturers by RSI sufferers, have developed new keyboards designed to eliminate the ergonomic problems of a traditional flat keyboard. Those problems can be significant for anyone suffering from RSI.

The flat keyboard tends to force the fingers to arch, creating tension in the back of the hand. In addition, the rectangular shape of the traditional keyboard causes the typist to hunch his shoulders and rotate the forearms inward. The QWERTY layout, which comes from the typewriter, was designed to slow down typists so that the basic mechanisms of the machine wouldn't be damaged by overly speedy typing. It succeeded in doing that, but it poses a risk to fingers and hands because it forces users to hit the shift key and common letters like "A" with the weakest finger, the pinkie.

Alternative keyboards are designed to address those problems. First and foremost, they are designed with the hands, not the mechanism of the machine, in mind. Working from the ergonomic theory that it is best to try to keep the hands in a neutral position rather than the traditional palms-down position used on flat keyboards, alternative keyboards come in a variety of shapes and sizes to permit hands to work from a comfortable position. They often look rather odd, but they're typically easy to use. (See Figure 5.3.)

Choosing a keyboard boils down to personal style and needs, according to David Thompson, Ph.D., a professor emeritus of industrial engineering at Stanford University and an ergonomics consultant. "The bottom line is that there is no one keyboard for everyone."

Three basic designs currently available are the split keyboard, which permits users to adjust the pieces to a comfortable width; split keyboard with a raised center, which eases ulnar deviation and some pronation; and the well keyboard,

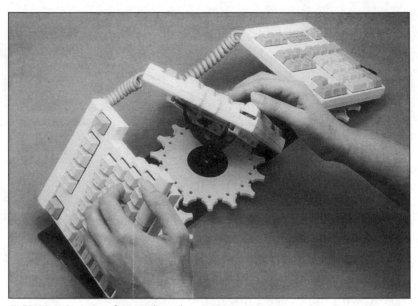

FIGURE 5.3: A Comfort Keyboard.
Reprinted with permisssion of Health Care Keyboard Company, Inc.

designed to eliminate the arching forced by flat keyboards by placing the keys in a well. There are other designs, such as the chord keyboards, where one or more keys are hit simultaneously, although the keyboards are not in common usage. As with any new product, the market continues to change. If you can afford it, you can even get a custom-made keyboard.

Some German studies indicate that splitting and angling the keyboard reduces muscle tension and fatigue. As previously mentioned in chapter 3, recent studies done by the National Institute of Occupational Safety and Health and Marquette University did not find that alternative keyboards prevent RSI. They did find, however, that alternative keyboards have a positive impact on posture. Some users swear by them. The important thing is that there is now a choice of affordable, ergonomic keyboards that are compatible with most computer systems.

The DVORAK keyboard tackles the problem of the QW-
ERTY keyboard layout. Studies have shown that most keystrokes—52 percent—on a traditional keyboard are done on
the upper row, with only 32 percent done on the home row.
Few words in English can be typed using the home row exclu-
sively. Because the extra reaching forced by the QWERTY keyboard can lead to strain, the DVORAK keyboard puts all five
vowels and the three most common consonants (T, H, and N)
on the home row. As a result, 70 percent of your keystrokes remain on the home row. The goal is less strain for hands.

The biggest obstacle to alternative keyboards is our own
resistance to change, says Chris Leick, of Health Care Keyboard Company in Wauwautosa, Wisconsin. "When the alternative keyboards first came out, people looked at them as if
they were science fiction," she says. "They're just now gaining
recognition."

Stanford's Thompson advises anyone buying a keyboard
to try it out for at least two weeks in order to get used to it. In
some ways, it's like breaking in a new pair of shoes. He points
out that for many people, typing is such a highly learned skill
that they don't even have to think about it. When you type on
a different style of keyboard, new muscle groups come into
play, others relax more, and you may even be a little sore. You
need a little time to adjust and get the feel of it. The payoff is
worth the effort because a good alternative keyboard will ease
or eliminate some of the postural stress problems that contribute to RSI.

People considering alternative keyboards also need some
coaching, Thompson says. The appearance of some of the keyboards turns off some people, as does having to make the effort to learn something new. It helps to have someone who
can help you set it up properly. Some companies actually have
"ergonomics rooms," where employees can try out a number
of keyboards. If you're motivated, it's really not that hard to

make the switch. Thompson has spoken to people with serious RSI injuries who switched to alternative keyboards and were thrilled. One, he says, compared it to "pouring warm water over your shoulders."

Those who want to try an alternative keyboard should consider some of the following factors suggested by Leick and Thompson:

- Does the company offer a tryout period after which you can return it without any obligation?
- If you are looking at a keyboard that has separate sections, are they adjustable to allow for a personal fit?
- If you are looking at an adjustable keyboard, can the numeric keypad be positioned to the left?
- Is there a timing device that reminds you to take a break?
- When you strike the keys, do you feel a slight release in pressure during the keystroke?
- Does the keyboard have function keys allowing programmable macros for commonly used functions?
- Has the keyboard been evaluated under work conditions?
- Is the keyboard compatible with major computer systems?
- Does the keyboard company provide technical assistance?
- Is there a warranty? If so, for how long?

Laptops

Laptop computers have become popular. According to Dataquest, a San Jose, California, market research firm specializing in technology-related products, almost ten million laptops and notebooks were sold in 1995 in the United States. They're portable, convenient, and easy to use. Unfortunately, their design is not ergonomic and because they're often used on the road, in hotels, airplanes, and other places that weren't designed with office ergonomics in mind, they can cause problems. They're small, which can force hands and arms into awkward postures.

That means being creative when using one on the road. If you're in a hotel, place it on the desk usually provided in hotel rooms, but you may need to sit on a telephone book to allow your arms to be basically parallel to the floor when typing. If you have RSI symptoms, you'll know pretty quickly whether you are working in a safe position.

Some people use a plug-in mouse to avoid using the touch pads or track balls that come with many laptops, although that's probably not a good idea. A mouse can force you to overreach with your arm, and excessive use of the mouse has been associated with problems.

If you're using a laptop in the air, try to get a bulkhead seat to gain a little more room. Pull down the window shade to cut down glare, and try to increase the font size so that you can stretch your arms out a little bit more while typing.

ACCESSORIES

With the new awareness of the dangers of keyboarding, a host of products aimed at preventing problems is being marketed. Several should be seriously considered, including if you want to prevent problems. One is a copyholder. Most office-supply stores sell them cheaply. It is easily attached to the side of the monitor and can go a long way toward easing neck and shoulder strain. Another option is a separate copy stand. The point is to avoid bending the neck for long periods. Positioning source documents was the subject of a 1996 University of Northern Iowa study, which found that documents placed flat on a table to either side of the keyboard produced the highest level of muscle tension. Placing the document on a copyholder so that the body, head, keyboard, and source document were aligned produced the least muscle tension.

The other accessory, cheap and widely available, is a wrist rest. It comes in a variety of shapes and sizes, but the best bet is to get one that is padded. A wrist rest can be useful because it can help keep wrists in a neutral position and prevent postures that lead to problems like carpal tunnel syndrome, for example. One caution: If the wrist rest isn't comfortable or helping to keep hands and wrists in a neutral position, don't use it. Wrist rests are still somewhat controversial, with some experts advising that they be used and others saying that they shouldn't, in part because such a wide variety is available. You may have to try out several before you find one that works for you.

If you choose to use armrests, some can be clamped onto the edge of a workstation.

If you're short, you should consider a footrest. It's important to be able to place feet flat while typing.

Those who frequently use a telephone on the job should have a headset. Cradling the telephone between the head and neck for long periods, especially while typing at a keyboard, can cause painful neck and shoulder problems, according to several occupational studies. Shoulder rests that cradle the receiver between the shoulder and ear are somewhat helpful, but a headset is better.

A range of software is available to minimize keystrokes without relying on embedded menus that require lots of mouse use. Avoid software that requires excessive mouse or cursor use; it's not only more wear and tear on your hands but it can also be frustrating and stressful to have to navigate a lot of menus.

Some software alerts users either visually on the monitor or with a sound or light that it's time to take a break from typing. It's commonly available, but it won't do you much good unless you pay attention to it!

⚘

POINTING DEVICES—
MICE AND TRACKBALLS

A recent Swedish study found that using a mouse more than six hours a week—that's right, a week—poses a risk for users. Other current studies have found physical complaints associated with mouse use is on the rise. Although it certainly does not look physically demanding, using a mouse is just that. You have to hold up your arm to use it and also make fine-motor movements to click, drag, and guide it to precise locations. With a track ball, you don't have to move the entire device to move the cursor, but it may force you to cock your wrist, placing additional strain on it.

Some computer mouses have a click-lock feature that permits you to click the button, release it, move the cursor, and click again, eliminating the static load on finger flexors that is caused by dragging. If it's not a feature of the mouse you use, you might be able to find software that has it. In addition, some feature additional buttons that can be programmed to double-click with just a single click.

Some manufacturers make pointing devices that can be used on either side of the keyboard, but, of course, most are right-handed. Because the numeric keypad is also usually on the right side, that increases the strain on your right hand. If you are left-handed, consider ordering a pointing device that can be used on the left side.

In choosing a mouse or track ball, try to select one that feels comfortable in your hand, as well as easy to use. In setting up your workstation, try to keep your mouse or track ball at the same level as the keyboard in order to avoid holding your arm out too far or bending your wrist excessively. A keyboard tray that has a mouse shelf extension is one way to achieve that.

When selecting a trackball, think about the specific tasks for which it will be used, such as the kinds of cursor movements required and the level of precision needed.

Quick Fixes

You don't necessarily have to buy a lot of expensive ergonomic equipment to make the necessary adjustments. Often, there are simple, quick fixes you can do on your own. Here are some suggestions from Dora Potter, of the Long Island-based consulting company Ergonomic by Design:

- To elevate your monitor to a more comfortable viewing angle, place books under it and/or a hardcover 2- to 3-inch loose-leaf binder (high end at the front) under it. (If more than one person is using the same monitor, you can buy an adjustable platform on which to place it so that each person can adjust the monitor to the appropriate height.)
- To make a copyholder, you can use a picture frame as an easel and place the copy on that. If you prefer a hanging document holder, secure a lightweight ruler

with tape or Velcro to the top right or left side of the monitor. Suspend the document with a clip—the big plastic kind—or tape.

- To make your chair fit you better, use seat cushions for elevation and/or a backrest. You can also tie or tape towels around the back of the chair to create better lumbar support.
- Adjust or remove chair arms if they are in the way of typing, or if they cause you to elevate your shoulders. Use towels or rubber foam to soften hard chair arms, as long as it doesn't raise your shoulders too high.
- Use a piece of plywood on top of a table or desk to create the depth needed for positioning a monitor directly in back of the keyboard.
- Roll up a soft winter scarf to keyboard level to make a wrist rest.
- If necessary, a stable center desk drawer can be used for the keyboard, which must be level with the front of the drawer so that there is no high or hard edge to interfere with reaching the keys. You have to do this carefully because if you pull the drawer out only partway, you could force your hands into an awkward posture.
- A clipboard placed under the corner of the keyboard, secured with Velcro or heavy-duty tape, will provide a mouse extension

OFFICE DESIGN

In designing an office to minimize stress to your muscles and tendons, three things should be considered: lighting, temperature, and noise.

Lighting should be situated in a way to reduce glare. Indirect lighting is one way to do this. While you work, there should be no distracting light within your visual field. Furniture color and tone should be selected with that in mind as well. Avoid high-contrast colors and fabrics in favor of colors of similar brightness. In addition, avoid using reflecting colors or materials on desk surfaces or office machines.

Putting many computers into one room can raise the office temperature because of the heat the machines generate, so it is important to keep the office well-ventilated. Working in a cold environment is not advisable because muscles and tendons tend to contract more in the cold. The working temperature should be as comfortable as possible.

Computers also tend to dry out the ambient air. Decreased humidity, along with the tendency of computer users to blink a little less, can cause your eyes to dry out. So it's also important to regulate office humidity.

Noise causes a great deal of stress to the muscles and tendons, often without your being aware of it. In addition to the physical stress, studies have indicated that noise contributes indirectly to emotional stress levels. It's advisable to try to keep the noise down in an office.

WORKING SENSIBLY

Working sensibly doesn't mean working less. Paying attention to how you work can go a long way toward preventing RSI. You can do three key things: Take breaks, vary your tasks, and listen to your body.

Take Breaks

One of the best things you can do for yourself is to take breaks. Studies have consistently shown that frequent, short rest breaks help prevent RSI and improve productivity. Taking frequent breaks is at odds with the typical office or factory setup where fifteen- to thirty-minute breaks are allowed every few hours. To give your body the rest it needs from any sustained, repetitive activity, you need to take frequent breaks. You don't even have to get out of your chair to take the break; simply pausing for a few minutes is important.

The development of RSI has been linked to continuing to work despite fatigue. Rest breaks, therefore, should be taken before you get tired, not afterward. Rigidly specified breaks are not the answer, researchers say; instead, workers should be allowed flexibility in how they're taken but should not be allowed to skip them altogether. On the whole, rest breaks appear to improve the quality and quantity of work output.

When working at any task, but particularly at one on a computer, it's easy to get caught up in it. That's why some people actually program their computers to remind them to take breaks. It's easy to do, and it can be a big help.

Vary Your Tasks

Studies have shown that workplaces that have reorganized jobs so that tasks are varied have significantly cut their rates of RSI. If there are easy ways for you to do that in your own job, it's important because it eases the constant stresses on your body, which come from doing one task again and again.

If you can take a break from the keyboard and make a

phone call instead, that's a way to vary your tasks. Sending out mail, filing papers, or organizing your work all may be ways to change your routine. It is a little irritating to have to interrupt a project you've been working on, but it is far more disheartening to be forced to stop because of pain.

Listen to Your Body

Professionals who treat RSI often tell patients, "Listen to your body!" That's easier said than done. Few of us know the specific symptoms of RSI, and they're easy to confuse with other, less debilitating problems. It isn't fair to chide someone for ignoring her symptoms when many doctors still don't know what those symptoms mean. The symptoms don't always show up gradually. Many RSI sufferers report that their symptoms flared up suddenly.

Here's a simple rule of thumb: If you feel pain while working, *stop*. Check it out. See a doctor.

Another rule of thumb: The earlier you catch RSI, the better off you'll be.

Don't accept your pain as part of the job, or as one of the signs of growing old. It may not be RSI. It could well be something completely unrelated, but you won't know unless you get it checked. There is no glory in working through pain.

❃

A WORD ABOUT EXERCISE AND STRETCHING

Numerous studies have documented the benefits of exercise. It helps relieve stress, improves circulation, and increases strength, muscle flexibility, and range of motion. All of the benefits are important in preventing RSI. In addition, exercise promotes better general health, and the healthier you are in general, the better you will feel.

Although some personal trainers like to cite the maxim, "no pain, no gain," that's not true with RSI. Just as it is unwise to work through pain, it is unwise to exercise through it. But a good exercise program can help keep RSI symptoms at bay.

Aerobic exercise can improve overall tone and general health when done regularly and properly. It can be particularly helpful for older people because of the muscle degeneration and reduced elasticity of tendons that come with age. Low-impact activities, such as swimming, race walking, or hiking, can provide a safe cardiovascular workout. (See chapter 8 for more on exercise.)

Several prominent specialists in the field of RSI treatment recommend doing simple stretches at your desk to prevent RSI. They argue that computer users are like athletes and should warm up before they start typing, as well as stretch their muscles throughout the day. However, a National Institute of Occupational Safety and Health review of physical exercises recommended for VDT operators found a number of problems in the recommended exercises. More than one-third of the exercises were conspicuous and potentially embarrassing to perform, and half would significantly disrupt the work routine. Perhaps more important, many of the exercises actually were contraindicated, posing potential safety hazards because they exacerbated the biomechanical stresses on the body.

Another study found that the benefits of incorporating exercises into rest breaks were modest. Although stretching can be important in rehabilitating injured muscles (as will be discussed in chapter 8), it may not prevent injury.

Before undertaking any kind of exercise, check with your doctor.

TYPING TECHNIQUE

In recent years, much has been made of how typing technique contributes to RSI. Some of this has been based on the study of musicians, whose technique may well contribute to injury. In general, it's best to try to avoid banging the keys and to avoid awkward reaches for them. If, for example, you need to use a function key that is located in a spot that forces you to reach way up or over with your little finger, try reprogramming one of your programmable keys to do that function. You can also save your hands and fingers by using macros to do several tasks that normally would require a number of keystrokes.

Most touch-typists have been taught to keep their hands in basically one position, using the home row keys as the base. That is helpful for typing speed because you don't have to look at the keyboard while typing, but it does tend to encourage you to angle your wrist and stretch your little finger when you have to press a distant key. Some specialists advise against this. Instead, they suggest moving your whole hand up to the distant key when you need to press it. This can be a little disorienting to a touch-typist, but it may help save your fingers.

Another frequent complaint of RSI sufferers is pain in the thumb. Again, touch-typists are taught to hit the space bar with their right thumb. To avoid overusing one thumb, it may make sense to try alternating thumbs when hitting the space bar.

These may seem like small steps, but given the fact that anyone who uses a keyboard more than a few hours a day is likely to hit tens of thousands of keystrokes, these small steps may prevent some of the debilitating tendon and muscle damage that result from overuse.

In using the mouse, people generally move it with just their wrist or with their entire arm. Positioning is important for the mouse because if it is poorly placed, you are likely to develop pain under your shoulder blade and down your arm. Keep it at roughly the same level as the keyboard and close by so that you don't have to reach up or out to use it. You can also cut down on mouse use by keeping your files in your computer in one easily accessible place. This can help you avoid undue shoulder stress and subsequent shoulder problems. In addition, try out the fit of a mouse before you select one; experts believe the size of the mouse in your hand can influence how hard you grip it and how often you click it.

All of these suggestions for preventing RSI may seem like a lot to think about, but once you have it down, you won't have to think much about it anymore. And ergonomic adjustments have solved many people's problems.

CHAPTER 6

DIAGNOSING RSI

✻

Rebecca, a writer in New York, can no longer do household chores like opening jars, carrying groceries, or doing dishes. Although she believes her condition is improving, she thinks that if she had known as much about RSI two years ago as she does now, she would have taken steps to protect herself. "The problem with RSI is you don't know you've hurt yourself until after you've done it," she says.

✻
GET TREATMENT EARLY

The most important piece of advice you can take from this book is something RSI sufferers, doctors, and therapists all agree on: *Get treatment early.*

The earlier you treat it, the better off you'll be. RSI develops slowly, over weeks, months, even years. Recovery from RSI can take as long, especially if you put off getting treatment. The sooner you catch it, the less time you'll spend in treatment.

It may be difficult to catch it early because you often don't know it's happening *while* it's happening. Some people still have difficulty believing they were injured by typing even after they experience burning arms and tingling hands.

One professional man, who prided himself on staying in shape and eating the right foods, was surprised to find that his elbows and wrists ached after he had spent hours night after night surfing the Internet. He said he couldn't believe typing could cause him that much pain—even though he had seen his wife forced out of work for several years because of a severe case of RSI. After several weeks of denying the possibility that he, too, could have RSI, he finally sought treatment and adjusted his workstation. The pain subsided.

He was lucky. He caught his RSI early. You can, too, if you pay attention to your body. Initially, the aches and pains of RSI can seem so innocuous that you may even feel as if you're whining if you mention them. Or you may think you don't type enough to get injured. Even if you rarely type, the amount of time you spend with your hands hovering over a keyboard composing a thought can be problematic because your muscles are still contracting to hold your arms in place—contributing to static muscle loading. You may be spending more time than you realize at activities that could put you at risk.

The point is that you need to be aware of the warning signs and get help if you have early symptoms. If you don't get it treated or make any change in the way you work, your injury will grow worse.

Don't let that happen to you. Pay attention to the warning signs:

Warning Signs

- Do you have occasional tingling in your hands or fingertips?
- Do you frequently massage your arms or hands to relieve tightness?
- Do your shoulders or neck constantly ache?
- Do you wake up at night with pain or tingling?
- Do your arms feel weak?
- Do you have difficulty gripping objects?
- Do your hands or arms feel sore even after you've stopped working?
- Do you have frequent headaches or feel tension in your neck and shoulders?
- Does your pain persist for twenty-four hours after you've stopped an activity?

If you have any of these symptoms, see a doctor. Don't write these off as a sign of aging or being out of shape. You may, in fact, be aging and out of shape, but you could still have RSI!

❧ FINDING A DOCTOR

Not every physician is familiar with RSI. Although the problem is widespread enough so that more and more health professionals are educated about it, there are still some doctors who insist it's a psychosomatic illness. The debate is raging, with a few particularly vocal proponents of the view that RSI victims are mainly malingerers who simply want to get out of work. Because RSI is complex and hard to diagnose, some physicians feel justified in taking that view. RSI is not as obvious as a broken bone, but it can be as crippling—or even more so in severe cases.

Melita, who worked as a production coordinator in a Minneapolis printing plant, recalls with some bitterness the trouble she had finding a sympathetic and knowledgeable doctor after she was injured in 1990. She was in pain for about nine months before she was finally diagnosed. "I got blown off by about five doctors," she says. "But I kept going until I found a doctor who knew what it was. By then, my hand had stopped functioning."

She eventually had two surgeries on her hands. She tried to return to work but couldn't handle it physically. Today, Melita is still so disabled she is unable to return to work. She finds simple tasks, like bagging her own groceries or flossing her teeth, impossible. Though angry about her experience, she said, "I'm going to continue living my life. I'm not going to let this get to me."

Although horror stories like Melita's abound, there are many competent and compassionate doctors who can treat RSI. One woman was so relieved after finding a doctor who listened to her and understood what she was talking about that she cried on her way out of his office. She later laughed at the memory, but said she had just been so happy that someone finally understood what she was going through.

A good doctor is critical to your recovery.

If you have a friend or acquaintance with RSI, ask her for a referral. Or, if you see a doctor for other reasons—like a gynecologist or dermatologist—ask her for a referral. Doctors frequently know the best people in their fields, and often, they'll tell you. Another great source of information are other health professionals—nurses, physical therapists, and occupational therapists—who work regularly with doctors and who will give you frank opinions. Don't be afraid to ask.

Certain medical specialties are more likely to be familiar with RSI. They include physiatrists, who are specialists in physical medicine and rehabilitation; occupational physicians, who focus on workplace illness and injuries; neurologists, who specialize in problems of the nervous system; orthopedists, who are surgically oriented specialists in the area of joints and bones; and sometimes, rheumatologists, who are concerned with tissue diseases, including arthritis.

If you don't have the name of a specialist, call your local medical association. It can tell you whether a physician or practice group is taking on new patients and whether the physician is board-certified, meaning he has passed rigorous tests in the field. If the medical society can't help, call the American Board of Medical Specialties to find out whether a particular doctor is board-certified. (See the appendix for the number.) Another source to check is *The Official ABMS Directory of Board Certified Medical Specialists*, which is available at many libraries.

You could call a doctor-referral service, but bear in mind that these services often charge a fee to list doctors and don't always screen the people they list. A better source might be to try your local hospital or medical society; they often have doctor-referral services. It can be a good starting point, so that you can get a few names to check further.

If you are inclined to do research, there are a number of RSI-related Websites on the Internet with the names of doctors. Reference articles in your local library can also lead you to a doctor.

A final resource is a local RSI support group. Such support groups are found worldwide. Often, they can provide names of doctors, even if they won't make specific recommendations. If you want to contact a support group in your area, check the appendix in the back of this book, which lists groups. Even if your area is not listed in the appendix, some of the larger groups know of contacts elsewhere.

In all likelihood, you won't have to look too far to find an educated, ethical, and experienced doctor. Patients learn pretty quickly, and word of mouth spreads fast. Try to get the names of more than one physician. Even if you have the names of several who are equally competent, there may be only one with whom you feel comfortable. And the key is to find a doctor with whom you feel comfortable.

Try to avoid the *mills* that make ethical doctors cringe, the medical practices in which unscrupulous doctors exaggerate a patient's condition for legal purposes. They see huge caseloads and generate huge incomes, but rarely are they said to provide good treatment to their patients. Anyone dealing with the worker's compensation system because of RSI wants a doctor to be an advocate. But a good doctor can be an advocate without exaggerating your claim.

In selecting a doctor, look for several important qualities.

1. *Does the doctor have expertise in the area?*
   Most doctors spend limited time studying soft-tissue injuries in medical school. In fact, RSI wasn't considered a major medical problem when most of today's physicians attended medical school. Because it can be difficult to diagnose, it's important to find someone with related clinical expertise. The doctor also should keep up with new developments in the field, which could make a difference in your treatment. In short, your doctor must have an understanding of the mechanisms of injury.

2. *Does the doctor listen to you?*
   Some doctors underestimate the importance of communication. A survey conducted by the American College of Physicians listed the key elements of high-quality patient care and asked both patients and physicians to rank them. Both groups picked clinical skills

as number one; but patients ranked communication as number two, while doctors ranked it sixth.

3. *Does the doctor explain things to you in an understandable fashion?*
   Sustaining an injury such as RSI can be a bewildering experience for you, your family, and your coworkers. To deal with it, you need to understand it. Any anxiety you feel will only be heightened if your doctor confuses you with obscure jargon.

4. *If your injury is work-related, is your doctor willing to do the necessary paperwork for worker's compensation?*
   Navigating the maze of worker's compensation is often confusing and frustrating. It is absolutely essential to have a doctor who is on your side, who is willing to file the necessary forms and appear at a hearing, if necessary. The paperwork of worker's compensation is a chore. In addition, worker's compensation usually doesn't pay doctors as well as private insurance does. If your employer decides to challenge your case, it can take months to get approval for treatment and/or payment for care. A doctor's frustration with the system is understandable, but you will not be able to get the care you need unless you have someone who is willing to deal with it.

5. *Do you feel comfortable with the doctor?*
   This is clearly very personal. Decide whether your doctor's style suits you. If your doctor seems distracted, dictatorial, or rushed, you may need to move on to someone else. Or, if the doctor views your injury with skepticism, you should consider going elsewhere. To be your advocate, your doctor must believe you.

In summing up what to look for, one point is key: Many doctors can make an isolated diagnosis, but it is important for your doctor to be able to do more than that. She must be able to pull together your work history, outside interests, and medical and family history and use the information to help determine the mechanism of injury. Treating only the symptoms, without understanding what caused your injury, doesn't do much good. If your doctor can understand and explain what caused your injury, you will be armed with the information you need to prevent recurrences or to at least handle them more effectively. Without that understanding, everyone winds up feeling frustrated and angry. With it, you can make strides toward getting better.

Once you find the right doctor, the real work begins.

✣
WHAT TO EXPECT IN YOUR FIRST DOCTOR'S VISIT

Your first visit with the doctor you have selected could set the tone for the rest of the relationship. Your doctor should listen to your complaints, take a complete medical, work, and personal history, do a thorough physical exam, and make a clear diagnosis.

Listening to Your Complaints

Going to a doctor can be a trying experience. After all, you are seeing a doctor because you are in pain and need help. You may be feeling overwhelmed and panicked. Your doctor should be sensitive to your fears and try to be reassuring. For your part, you need to do what you can to help your doctor understand your problem.

When talking about your physical complaints, be thorough. Try to describe them in as specific a manner as possible. Saying only that, "my arm hurts," is not nearly as helpful as saying, "I feel a shooting pain from the underside of my wrist up my forearm." If you have difficulty finding the right words to describe your pain, mention the activities you have trouble doing. It may be hard for you to open a jar or grasp objects. If that's the case, tell your doctor so.

Though some doctors think RSI patients exaggerate their pain, it is probably more likely that they're *minimizing* it. Because it can be a frightening injury, it is common for patients to be in denial about the problem. Denial is a universal emotional defense, and sometimes, it's appropriate. But it's risky with RSI. If the pain burns, admit it. Don't worry about looking like a whiner or malingerer. This is not a time to be stoic. You cannot expect people to read your mind or feel your pain. One occupational therapist routinely has her patients circle words from a long list of adjectives that best describe their pain. She recalls being stunned the day one patient told her that her pain was not too bad and then circled words like *burning* and *stabbing*.

At the same time, you are likely to have more success with your doctor if you use a businesslike tone. In a recent study conducted at the Walter Reed Army Medical Center in Washington, D.C., forty-four internists were split into groups and shown a video of the same woman describing her symptoms. In one video, she was dressed conservatively and spoke in a businesslike manner. In the other, she wore flashy clothes and jewelry and spoke histrionically. The study concluded that the woman's demeanor affected the physicians's diagnoses. Seventy-three percent of those who viewed the emotional performance offered diagnoses of panic attacks or anxiety. In contrast, fewer than one-third who viewed the other video suspected anxiety.

Your doctor probably will ask you many questions that should help you describe your problem more clearly. Your doctor should respect confidentiality, so don't withhold information. It's in your best interest to provide all the information you can. It's necessary to rule out anything that might complicate your case, like diabetes.

Some questions you may be asked include the development and frequency of the symptoms and/or pain, quality of the pain, and intensity of the pain. Sometimes, a doctor will ask you to rate your pain on a scale of one to ten. And some doctors may provide you with what's called a *pain drawing* to help you better describe your pain. In addition, your doctor should ask you what activities make your pain better or worse. (See Figure 6.1.)

If you find your doctor interrupting you and acting impatient, politely ask your doctor to listen until you finish. (That's tough to do, however. Most people don't like it when people point out their rude behavior!) If the doctor persists in interrupting you, consider finding another one.

Don't let any doctor act as if you are too stupid to understand the complexities of the human body. This is especially important if you are deemed a candidate for surgery. You must understand the procedure and whether there are possible complications. If you have any misgivings about surgery or your doctor, don't submit to surgery. And beware of anyone who wants to schedule surgery immediately.

Remember: You are the consumer. It is part of your doctor's job to listen to you and treat you with respect.

Taking Your History

Because it is essential to rule out underlying conditions that may be similar to or contribute to RSI, a good doctor will take a thorough medical, work, and social history. A thorough history will also help determine the severity of the problem, the specific type or types of RSI, and the site of the injury.

If your doctor uses a questionnaire, it should include questions about which hand is dominant; any recent changes you have experienced in activities or on the job; when your pain or discomfort started; how long it has been bothering you; and whether the pain stays in one place or radiates. Figure 6.1 lists some of the additional questions developed by Craig H. Rosenberg, M.D., a physiatrist who specializes in RSI, among other things.

The Physical Exam

A physical exam can be an unnerving experience, especially for someone suffering from RSI. It's no fun to be poked, prodded, and asked all sorts of personal questions. It's particularly hard on someone with RSI because the physical exam may cause you pain the next day. Don't be afraid to tell a doctor to be gentle; you are the one who has to live with the pain.

The physical exam is likely to include looking for outward signs of injury; checking range of motion; palpation to check for tenderness, pain and/or trigger points; examining your posture; and measuring strength.

Outward signs of injury   These include such things as ganglion cysts, swelling, and muscle atrophy. Weakened or injured muscles can atrophy quickly.

Range of motion   You will probably be asked to move your arms up, down, and out to the side. Similar tests will be done on your neck and wrists. Most people with RSI are so focused on their pain that they are surprised to find out just how limited their range of motion has become. Normally, you should

PATIENT PAIN FORM

Name: _____ Date: _____

Where is your pain now?
Mark the areas on your body where you feel the sensations described below, using the appropriate symbol. Mark the areas of radiation. Include all affected areas. To complete the picture, please draw in your face.

Aching	Numbness	Pins and needles	Burning	Stabbing
▲ ▲ ▲	■ ■ ■	● ● ●	◆ ◆ ◆	○ ○ ○

Right   Left   Left   Right

How bad is your pain now?
Please mark with an X on the body where the pain is worst now.

Describe your pain. (This may be accompanied by a pain drawing.)

How often does your pain occur?
○ constantly (more than 75% of day)
○ frequently (50 to 75% of day)   ○ occasionally
○ varies unpredictably   ○ intermittently

How long do symptoms last?
○ minutes   ○ hours   ○ days

When is the pain typically worse?
○ morning   ○ afternoon   ○ evening   ○ after waking up
○ no relationship to the time of day

FIGURE 6.1: Patient Pain Form.

List the major activities the pain prevents you from doing.
Which of the following affects your pain? (Mark "B" for conditions that make the symptoms better and "W" for worse for those that exacerbate it, and leave blank for no effect.)

__ anger	__ running	__ writing
__ anxiety	__ household chores	__ shaking hands
__ reaching	__ intercourse	__ squeezing objects
__ carrying objects	__ grooming	__ standing
__ weather	__ opening doors	__ strain/stretch
__ deadline	__ opening bottle/jar	__ stress
__ doing buttons	__ overwrought	__ sleeping
__ dressing	__ personal care	__ sitting
__ driving	__ pick up keys/pens	__ tension
__ exercise	__ heat	__ typing
__ fatigue	__ rubbing	__ walking
__ grabbing	__ reading (holding book or paper)	

Which of the following leisure activities do you participate in and for how many hours per week? If you check one, describe the activity and how long you have been doing it.

- ○ gardening _____
- ○ woodworking _____
- ○ auto mechanics _____
- ○ knitting/crocheting _____
- ○ play musical instrument _____
- ○ glass etching _____
- ○ golf _____
- ○ tennis/racquetball _____
- ○ bowling _____
- ○ shooting _____
- ○ sports _____
      which sport(s) _____
- ○ weightlifting _____
- ○ sailing _____
- ○ bike riding _____
- ○ home-computer use _____
- ○ other activities _____

Do you drive a car?
   ○ yes   ○ no

If yes, what kind of car do you usually drive?
   ○ standard   ○ automatic

Is the steering wheel adjustable?
   ○ yes   ○ no

Is the seat adjustable?
   ○ yes   ○ no

FIGURE 6.1: Patient Pain Form, *continued overleaf*

Medical History

Do you have or have you had any of the following?

○ arthritis	○ coronary disease	○ leukemia
○ allergies	○ diabetes	○ ulcers
○ asthma	○ epilepsy	○ pneumonia
○ bleeding tendency	○ hypertension	○ tuberculosis
○ cancer	○ jaundice	○ thyroid
○ cardiac problems	○ kidneys	○ anxiety
○ depression	○ other _____	

Occupational History

Please provide your current job description. Include how long you have been working at this position and describe previous positions. _____

What equipment do you use? _____

Check any of the conditions applicable to you:

    ○ deadlines   ○ taking notes

    ○ a lot of time on the phone   ○ use of computer/typewriter

    ○ use of repeated keys on the computer/typewriter, etc.

    ○ use of particular function keys on a regular basis

       specify: _____

    ○ other conditions or functions you consider important: _____

    _____

Describe your daily work activities _____

_____

_____

Please indicate the following:

Hours a day spent using keyboard or other equipment	_____
Average hours worked per week	_____
Amount of overtime per week	_____
If appropriate, words per minute typed	_____
Description of pen used	_____
Type of word processing system	_____
Keyboard type	_____
Other significant activities	_____

Does your job require:

    ○ bending   ○ carrying   ○ lifting   ○ pulling

    ○ reaching   ○ stretching   ○ standing   ○ sitting

If you checked any of the above activities, please describe them.

_____

_____

_____

FIGURE 6.1: Patient Pain Form, *continued*

be able to bend your wrist up to eighty degrees; for many people with RSI, that's simply impossible. One woman with rotator cuff tendinitis was shocked to discover that she couldn't lift her right arm above her shoulder. Only then, she said, did she realize she had a serious problem that needed to be treated.

Palpation The physician will likely press different spots on your hands, arms, and shoulders to locate areas of tenderness or pain. She also may ask you to open and close your hands to see if you feel pain upon making that movement. The doctor should check for trigger points, which are painful nodules—or knots—that are probably caused by stress on the muscle. They are easy to find: When pressed, they can cause a great deal of pain in that spot or refer it to another part of the body. The doctor should also check for crepitus, which is indicated by a crackling or crunching over the joints and tendons upon examination, and for evidence of tendon thickening.

Posture Your doctor will probably check your posture. Sometimes bad posture becomes such a habit that it is actually a postural dysfunction, which is hard to change. It's important to take note of it, as it can be a key diagnostic clue. Tightness in the pectoralis minor muscle in the chest, for example, can indicate thoracic outlet syndrome.

Strength Your doctor should test your strength by asking you to do simple resistance exercises, like pressing your hand and/or fingers against her hand. The doctor may ask you to squeeze an instrument called a dynamometer, which measures the number of pounds you can pull. Another test requires that you squeeze a pinch meter as hard as you can in order to measure hand and finger strength. You may also be tested for balanced forearm strength.

Don't be surprised if the doctor performs these tests more than once during the examination and in subsequent examinations. Many factors, such as fatigue, handedness (meaning which hand is dominant), time of day, age, nutritional state, pain, and the patient's cooperation, can influence the outcome of such tests, according to the American Medical Association's *Guides to Evaluation of Permanent Impairment.* Usually, tests to measure grip and pinch strength are given three times with each hand at different times.

If only one hand is injured, the measurements are averaged and then compared with the measurements taken from the other hand in order to make a comparison of normal pinch and grip strength. If both hands are injured, the measurements are averaged and compared with average normal strengths. These average normal strengths have been calculated based on several factors, including age and occupation. For men, average normal grip strength is 47.6 in the dominant hand, and 45 in the nondominant hand. For women, it is 24.6 in the dominant hand, and 22.4 in the nondominant hand.

If you are acutely inflamed, you really don't want to do these tests because you'll pay the price in pain hours later. The tests can wait until your pain has dissipated.

Many doctors are familiar with the techniques used to test for carpal tunnel syndrome, and it's likely you'll go through those as well. They include the Phalen's test, Tinel's sign, and testing for fingertip sensation.

Phalen's test   This test calls for you to hold the back of your hands together with your fingers pointing downward for up to one minute. You will be asked if you feel any tingling in your fingertips. If you do, it is an indication that you may have carpal tunnel syndrome.

Elbow hyperflexion   This test involves bending your elbow and is used to test for ulnar-nerve entrapment at the elbow.

Tinel's sign   In this test the doctor taps the area over the median nerve on the palm side of your hand and asks you if you feel tingling afterward. If you do, it is another indication that you may have carpal tunnel syndrome.

Fingertip sensation   There are two methods commonly used to test the sensation in your fingertips. In one, you are asked to close your eyes while the doctor holds an instrument that looks like a tiny pizza wheel against your finger. You will be asked whether you feel one point or two. Some doctors use a pin to test fingertip sensation. In the other test, you again are asked to keep your eyes closed while the doctor brushes your fingertip with a long filament and asks whether you can feel it. These tests are used to determine if you have lost sensation in your fingertips, which can be another indicator of carpal tunnel syndrome or other nerve entrapment.

Reflex testing   Most people have had their reflexes checked as a matter of routine in a doctor's office. It is done here to rule out cervical radiculopathy, which is simply carpal tunnel syndrome of the neck (the median nerve is compressed at the neck).

Electrodiagnostic tests   Many doctors recommend electrodiagnostic testing, which includes an electromyogram, or EMG, and other nerve-conduction tests. Electrodes are used to determine how fast your nerves conduct nerve impulses. If there is slowing, it is generally considered to be a positive sign of carpal tunnel syndrome. Nerve-conduction tests can be useful because they can help a physician decide on a course of treatment for symptoms of trapped nerves, such as those common with carpal tunnel syndrome. An EMG is not foolproof, however. One recent study found false positives in up to 27 percent of EMGs conducted. The experience of the physician conducting the test is important.

Those tests are not conclusive, however, because other conditions can mimic the symptoms of carpal tunnel syndrome. Additional testing, such as X rays or blood work, may be required to rule them out or pin them down. For example, symptoms of Lyme disease can appear similar to those of RSI, which is why it's so important for your doctor to look at the whole picture. A good doctor is a good detective.

Diagnosis

After the exam, the doctor should be able to offer a fairly specific diagnosis. That's important because although there are general considerations in the treatment of RSI, specific problems require specific modalities. Thoracic outlet syndrome would be treated differently from carpal tunnel syndrome, for example.

A specific diagnosis is also important to establish whether your RSI is work-related. If it is, you are probably eligible for worker's compensation to pay for your visits to your doctor and physical or occupational therapist, if therapy is prescribed. Worker's compensation will also pay for at least part of your lost income if you are forced out of work by your injury. If you get the wrong diagnosis, it could have serious financial consequences.

Finally, knowing your diagnosis helps you know what to expect and how to deal with your RSI. If you are diagnosed with carpal tunnel syndrome, you will understand why you might wake up at night with shooting pains in your hands and arms. Or, if you are diagnosed with shoulder tendinitis, you can probably expect pain to result from any large, overhead movements of your shoulder. Labeling the problem is the first step toward managing it.

A good diagnosis should tell you what body parts are affected, the degree of impairment you have suffered, and the likely cause. It will also tell you whether you have a chronic injury. From the doctor's point of view, it helps to identify the appropriate treatment or intervention.

After the initial exam, a relationship begins—your relationship with your doctor.

❈
WORKING WITH YOUR DOCTOR

Generally, there are no quick fixes when it comes to treating RSI. If you're lucky, you may be able to ease your discomfort with some ergonomic changes to your workstation. If you have more than a mild injury, however, you will have to spend time and effort working at your recovery. That is why you must build a relationship with your doctor because you'll likely be seeing him more than once. It could be as little as a few visits over four to six weeks for a mild case, or it could be many visits over the course of a year (or more) for a severe, chronic case. There is no average number of visits because each case varies. Though you may feel overwhelmed and panicked by your pain, you cannot afford to be a passive consumer. It's *your* body and *your* health. Take charge of it and work with your doctor.

Once you find a doctor who listens to you and who is reassuring, as well as realistic about your case, be sure to hold up your end of the bargain.

Be responsible about your care. Be punctual for appointments. If you are constantly late to appointments or forget about them altogether, ask yourself why. Be honest about smoking, diet, and alcohol consumption and whether you take medication as prescribed. You cannot expect a doctor to be able to diagnose you accurately if you're not being completely honest with him.

Ask questions. If you need a reminder, make a list before your appointment. It's easy to get caught up in talking about one problem and wind up forgetting about another question you have. Or you simply may feel too panicked by the pain to remember to ask everything. A good doctor will take the time to answer all your questions. Use your time with your doctor to obtain the information you need, in particular, to identify which activities make your symptoms worse. Often, a good doctor can help you do that simply by listening and asking questions.

Don't let anyone dismiss you. RSI sufferers often complain that doctors don't believe they have a real problem. A librarian recalls bitterly the first time she saw a doctor for her pain, which was so bad she was dropping books. She had been unable to see her regular doctor because he was booked, so she took the first available appointment with another doctor. After he examined her, he told her, "You've got that fashionable disease." She tried to go back to work one-handed, but eventually, she couldn't use her hand at all. By then, she was able to get an appointment with her regular doctor, who was considerate and thorough. He pulled her out of work immediately.

Sometimes it may be a problem with a member of the doctor's staff. One RSI patient was stunned when a secretary insisted that she fill out a long medical form months after she had begun treatment, even though the secretary knew the woman was so disabled she couldn't write. The secretary then made a sarcastic remark about the patient's slow recovery. Furious, the patient told her quietly she had no business commenting on her recovery and complained to the doctor. The doctor was sympathetic, and the secretary never made any more comments.

Think about your own expectations. If you want your doctor to take your phone calls immediately, you should expect that your own office visits will be interrupted by calls from other patients. If you want your doctor's undivided attention, you should also expect to wait for your calls to be returned.

Remember, you and your doctor are partners in your recovery. If you expect to be treated with respect, you need to treat your doctor and his staff with respect. They are there to help you.

❧ CHRONIC INJURY

In some cases, because it takes so long to develop RSI and because most people don't even feel the damage while it's occurring, RSI becomes a chronic injury. That means you'll be dealing with it for a fairly long time. It also means you'll be dealing with your doctor and other health professionals on your case for a while.

Chronic pain can cause shaky relationships, not only with your loved ones but with your doctor and other health professionals. It's much easier for a health professional to deal with acute pain—it can be diagnosed and fixed fairly readily. Chronic pain is much harder, and often patients with it find themselves caught up in a maze of misdiagnoses.

To feel constant pain is a depressing, frustrating experience. You may well be angry if you don't see immediate improvement. But remember, your doctor and therapists want to see you get better. They may feel just as frustrated if you don't improve. If you have chronic pain, you and your doctor must be prepared to deal with it over the long term. However, not every health professional is prepared to do that. If your doctor or therapist isn't, find someone who is.

This is not to say that you should start "doctor-shopping," which is the term physicians use for patients who bounce from one doctor to another. Searching for the one doctor who has the cure will be fruitless and frustrating. Doctors and therapists are wary of patients who complain of having seen a lot of medical professionals, without results.

One woman who had painful shoulder tendinitis was so angry that her job had caused her injury that she took it out on every physical therapist who worked with her. She demanded special treatment in private rooms and then refused to do the prescribed exercises because she found them "boring." Eventually, no physical therapist wanted to work with her, and the less-senior people who ended up treating her gave her only cursory care.

Once you find a doctor who understands your problem, you must help him treat you by following his advice. It's not uncommon to hear health professionals talk about patients who complain bitterly about their problems yet fail to follow medical advice. Then there are others who think they know more than their doctor and simply ignore what they're told. Presumably, you are seeing a doctor because you want to get better. Do what you're told! You cannot expect to be taken seriously unless you take your treatment seriously.

Treatment for RSI can be a bewildering experience. It's not just a matter of going to a doctor and getting a prescription for pain pills. It often involves other specialists.

CHAPTER 7

YOUR TREATMENT TEAM

Lorraine, a staff analyst in New York, first noticed a problem with her hands when her handwriting started to deteriorate. She joked about it, telling friends that the better educated a person was, the worse their handwriting seemed to be. She didn't let it interfere with her work, which consisted of spending a great deal of time at a computer terminal designing spread sheets and doing computer analyses.

Then one day, she woke up with pain so severe she couldn't move her right hand. It was locked. She was able to pry it open with her other hand; she called a hand doctor, who advised her to get a splint. That didn't seem to help, but she says, "I thought, 'Oh, I'll go to the doctor once or twice and I'll be fine.'"

That was in 1995. Since then, Lorraine has been thrust into a maelstrom of worker's compensation, charges of employment discrimination, and ongoing occupational therapy. Her injury was so severe that for a while, she couldn't even brush her teeth. The pain was so bad and the stress so great at work, Lorraine says, she was forced to take early retirement from a job she wanted to keep. Though her condition has improved somewhat, she still copes with pain and physical limitations. "It's hard enough to deal with the pain," she says. "You don't know, will it go away?"

❧ TREATMENT TAKES TIME

For most people, the pain, weakness, and loss of functioning caused by RSI will disappear. But Lorraine's story illustrates something many RSI patients don't understand initially: When you start treatment, *be prepared for the long haul.*

In the worst cases, treatment can take weeks, months, even years. That may be hard to believe, but remember, it took weeks, months, and possibly years for the injury to develop.

Healing takes time. Researchers don't know yet why it takes tissues that are torn, as is often the case in RSI, so long to heal. Part of it may be due to the fact that tensed, injured muscles don't receive the oxygen and other nutrients needed for healing because of reduced blood circulation. Another factor in more serious injuries may be the formation of scar tissue, which interferes with surrounding muscle, causing more microtears and even more scar tissue.

Don't let the prospect of long-term treatment depress or scare you. It's not easy, to be sure. At times, it can be frustrating, even infuriating. But taken a day at a time, it can be done. And the time you take to heal may open up new opportunities for you. As Lorraine says, "I think positive things can come out of the negative."

YOUR TREATMENT TEAM

RSI is not merely a physical problem. Because our hands are so central to who we are and what we do, the effects of RSI can be far-reaching. It affects your health, family, and work. It can shatter relationships you once took for granted, wreak havoc on your financial security, and alter your perspective of the world. All that may sound dramatic, but it's not overstating the case.

It's essential to have a coordinated treatment "team." The standard medical model is not sufficient to treat RSI. It is not enough for a doctor to tell you to find a physical therapist, write out a prescription, and tell you to come back in a few months. "It's a jungle out there in terms of getting treatment that will help," says Rebecca, who was injured in 1995 and feels that her condition grew worse after seeing a doctor because she got so little concrete guidance. "My doctor made efforts to warn me, but I still did not comprehend that if I did not modify my work habits dramatically, I would be crippled for life."

In short, you need support. You need to know how to find the people who can help you deal with problems as they arise and help you change your work habits, as well as other activities. Your team may consist of a doctor and physical therapist, or it may include other professionals, such as an occupational therapist, psychotherapist, ergonomist, and vocational rehabilitation specialist. It's unlikely that you'll find everyone you need under one roof, although that would be ideal.

It all begins with your doctor.

Your Doctor

As the person in charge of your treatment, it's up to your doctor to point you in the right direction. She also should lead the treatment team, be available to take calls from therapists, and review your progress with them. Many doctors don't do that, however. They leave it up to the patient to navigate the medical maze, which can be mystifying to the uninitiated. Many doctors, so familiar with the medical world themselves, fail to realize that starting on a course of treatment, such as physical therapy, and learning how to cope with your injury are huge adjustments. Even intelligent people can be bewildered and, at times, overwhelmed. It's not realistic to expect every patient to know how or where to get help.

A knowledgeable, caring doctor will try to help you find the proper treatment and then monitor it carefully. It's your job as a patient to keep your doctor informed of what you're doing. One woman chose not to tell her doctor that she had decided to put her arms in slings because, "he doesn't do anything for me anyway. I just need him to write prescriptions." She liked the sympathy the slings elicited, but friends noticed that her arms seemed to get weaker. The slings meant that she rarely used her arms; and when she did, she had trouble with even the simplest of tasks, like carrying a plate of food. Whenever she saw her doctor, she took off the slings. She never told him about them and could not understand his confusion over her physical deterioration.

It's also important to tell your doctor about the problems RSI are causing you. There may be a simple solution to a problem that has been vexing. Or, if the problems are more interpersonal, your doctor may be able to recommend a professional who can help you. Some patients bristle at the suggestion of psychological counseling, as if it is meant to suggest that the injury is psychosomatic. However, if you are experiencing emotional distress because of your injury—and most people do—a qualified therapist may be able to help you through it.

In short, your doctor should be actively involved in your case. Anyone who isn't is doing you a disservice.

Your Physical Therapist

As part of your treatment, your doctor may decide that you need to see a physical and/or occupational therapist.

A physical therapist focuses on helping you reduce your pain, restore strength and mobility, and prevent the further loss of function. This may entail deep-tissue massage, use of hot and cold treatments, electric stimulation, and passive and active exercise. In a typical session, your therapist will use various treatment modalities and then guide you in exercises. Depending upon your injury, the exercises will vary.

Your therapist is also likely to give you a home program of exercises. It's not enough to simply attend therapy sessions; you need to follow through on your therapist's instructions. Treatment is not passive. You have to be actively involved in your recovery. That means doing any home program of exercises a therapist tells you to do. They may be boring, but they will help you. Again, it is essential that you take responsibility for your health.

An occupational therapist may also do massage but focuses on helping a patient who is disabled with work tasks and day-to-day living. The orientation is more functional. If, for example, writing causes you pain, to ease it an occupational therapist might suggest a different way to hold a pen. Or the therapist might suggest putting a thick grip on the pen. A good occupational therapist can find many creative ways to help you do things that may seem daunting because of the pain they cause. She can also recommend adaptive aids that make tasks easier.

An occupational therapist also can design a splint for you. Some doctors recommend using splints on a limited basis to help you accomplish tasks that might otherwise leave you in pain for a while. Miriam, for example, has carpal tunnel syndrome and works in a bookstore in Minneapolis. She wears splints whenever she has to shelve or carry books for any length of time. However, it is not recommended that you wear splints around the clock. (More on that will be discussed in the next chapter.)

A lot of therapists will say they know how to treat RSI. If your doctor has not recommended a specific therapist, ask any prospective therapist how many cases of RSI he has treated. Because you will be seeing this person on a regular basis, the office should be easily accessible. It's not worthwhile to travel many hours to a therapist who has a great reputation if that travel takes a toll on your body.

Most important is the rapport you feel with your therapist. You will likely be seeing that person two or three times a week for an extended period of time. Your therapist will know your hands, arms, and shoulders better than your doctor and should be making regular, written reports to your doctor about your progress. Your therapist should also have a sense of what kinds of things set you back, as well as how to motivate you when you are distressed by a setback. And your therapist should teach you how to handle any recurrence of pain and prevent it altogether.

Not every therapist likes to deal with a chronic injury. It's easier to work with a broken limb. They know more about what to do, and they see results more quickly. When your job is to help someone heal, it can be frustrating when it doesn't seem to be happening. Some therapists may feel like a failure if no progress is made. As a patient, be sure you have a therapist who is willing to stick it out.

Your Psychotherapist

Not everyone will want to see a psychotherapist. The root of your problem is, after all, physical. But a vicious cycle can start—the pain of RSI leads to emotional stress, which leads to muscle tension, which leads to more pain. Dealing with the emotional stress of the injury may help you reduce the pain. Again, the emotional distress is not the cause, it is merely part of the problem.

It would be difficult not to feel upset and angry. Your injury is painful, limiting, and frightening. And if you are dealing with the worker's compensation system, you are likely to be feeling frustrated and angry as well. You may find that you want to talk to someone who can help you with your feelings, or you may want to participate in an RSI support group. Not every psychotherapist understands chronic pain and injury or is even sympathetic to it. Again, if your doctor cannot provide you with a specific recommendation, choose a therapist carefully.

The psychotherapist you choose may be a clinical social worker, psychologist, or psychiatrist. Many psychotherapists have specialties, including dealing with chronic pain or injury. While that may be preferable, it may not be easy to find. More important is whether you trust and feel comfortable with the psychotherapist.

A good psychotherapist should be informed and flexible enough to use a range of psychotherapeutic models in treatment. The psychotherapist should have a sincere desire to help you, as well as enough intuition to communicate that he genuinely understands your experience. Your therapist should also be able to take criticism without retaliating. She should also be able to gently confront you in instances where you have made mistakes. Finally, she should be emotionally involved but still be able to maintain a degree of emotional distance.

Your Ergonomist

A personal ergonomist is a luxury few people have. Businesses, however, sometimes hire ergonomic consultants for office or plant redesigns. If you're fortunate enough to be able to consult with one, take advantage of the opportunity. An ergonomic consultant can help you make changes in your workstation that can help you prevent further pain and injury.

Unfortunately, many people claim to be experts in ergonomics but aren't. The title *ergonomist* is a relatively new one, although industrial engineers have been doing similar work for years. An ergonomist blends a variety of disciplines to make the work environment accommodate people, not the other way around.

When trying to find an ergonomist, ask about training, qualifications, and certification. To be certified with the Board of Certification in Professional Ergonomics, a person must have a master's or the equivalent in ergonomics or a related discipline and four years of full-time experience in the field, as well as submit a work product in ergonomic design to the board, and then take a seven-hour exam. It is also wise to ask about experience because ergonomists have a wide range of specialties. An ergonomist may have great technical expertise but not in the area you need. Also ask whether the ergonomist has consulted for any companies; that can give you a quick idea of a person's experience.

The Human Factors and Ergonomics Society (see listing in appendix) publishes a directory of ergonomic consultants, which lists their specialties and credentials. You also might find an ergonomist in your area by calling a local large company and asking whether they've used an ergonomist.

Professionals caution against listening to sales pitches of people trying to sell ergonomic products or people without formal training. Although the principles of ergonomics are simple, some people oversimplify them. The key is to adapt your workstation to *your* needs. It's essential to get this right.

Your Vocational Rehabilitation Counselor

Most people with RSI probably will never need a vocational rehabilitation counselor, but if you are seriously injured, you may. Many insurance companies will pay for counselors to assist people who are on disability return to work. Many states also provide vocational rehabilitation counseling free of charge. Their assistance can be helpful—from ideas on how to manage doing your job, to providing equipment you need to do it, and counseling.

Some insurance companies will pay for retraining for another career. This is another area where a vocational rehabilitation counselor can be of assistance.

Bear in mind that a counselor employed by an insurance company is eager to get you back to work to save the insurance company money. That is not to say that you should ignore the counselor's advice, but you should remember there may be options available to you other than those recommended. A counselor from a state vocational rehabilitation department works for a neutral agency and should be interested in your goals. Any counselor should be willing to consult with your doctor to help work out what's best for you.

When seeing a vocational counselor, you may be asked to take a test designed to discern your interests and skills. It can be an illuminating experience and may open up new possibilities to you.

Because it is important that your counselor thoroughly

understand your physical limitations, he may recommend a functional capacity exam, which is designed to identify your physical abilities by testing major motor strength and capacity. Such an exam can give your counselor—and your doctor— guidance about the kind and how much work you can do. After you complete the exam, your counselor should go over the results with you.

If necessary, a counselor will help you contact potential employers, as well as determine a strategy for getting a job. If you need it or want it, your counselor may even attend job interviews with you to explain your disability to a potential employer.

Most importantly, your counselor should be available to talk over any difficulties you've had in getting back to work or making a job change. He should be able to understand what you're going through and provide moral support. Studies have shown that as a rule, disabled workers are highly motivated workers; but the adjustment of returning to work with physical limitations can be difficult.

No Easy Answers

You may feel bewildered at this point, especially since your problem is still not understood by some members of the medical community. Indeed, you may not need all these professionals to help you deal with your RSI. However, RSI is a complex problem without easy answers. It may not be enough simply to consult with a doctor. Most of the time with RSI, the more help you can get, the better off you'll be.

If your doctor cannot provide recommendations for specialists, find the help you need yourself. A wide array of resources is available. You'll find that you'll need the support. And, as with any serious disease or injury, take it one day at a time.

GOAL OF TREATMENT

The goal of any treatment is simple—to enable you to get on with your life without reinjury and to stem your pain. (A range of standard treatment options will be discussed in the next chapter.) But the first issue to address is pain.

Physiology of Pain

One of the immediate goals you and your doctor will seek to accomplish in any course of treatment is to alleviate your pain. There are a number of ways to do this, but first, it's important to understand pain itself.

The classic explanation of pain is the stimulus-response concept: You are injured, and a message is relayed to the brain. The theory assumes that the intensity of pain is directly related to the severity of the injury and does seem to explain straightforward injuries. But this theory doesn't explain what is happening in the body when the injury isn't obvious, and when the pain persists over a long period.

A more recent view of pain presents it as a complex web of pain signals. One theory, called "imprinting," suggests that pain literally gets stamped onto the nervous system, which retains a memory of it even after the injurious activity has been stopped. Though it is not clear why this happens, one idea is that a disruption occurs in the balance of neurochemical transmitters, which can act either as painkillers or pain pro-ducers. Imprinting helps explain why pain may persist even after surgery eliminates the cause.

A related notion is that pain does not travel a one-way route, as suggested by the stimulus-response theory, but that there is continuous feedback between the brain and the in-jured area, and that the pain signal can be changed in the course of that feedback.

Finally, there is a phenomenon called "referred pain," in which the injury is in one part of your body, but the pain is in another. It is not uncommon, for example, to feel pain in your hand when a nerve in your neck is irritated. Sometimes the pain is not felt in the injured area. This may be puzzling and cause you to doubt your physician, but it happens frequently. Trigger points are often the source of referred pain in people with RSI.

These theories have led to a number of approaches to pain, ranging from the simple to the sophisticated. Not every approach is appropriate for every case. Specific injuries re-quire specific treatments. But the following are some of the ways physicians treat pain. Most are done under the guidance of a physical or occupational therapist.

Psychogenic Pain

Sometimes, when a doctor is unable to pinpoint the cause of your pain—a fairly frequent occurrence with RSI—she may label the pain "psychogenic," which means "of mental or emo-tional origin." In other words, it's all in your head.

Although psychogenic pain is real and it is important not to minimize pain that is emotionally based, RSI pain is not psychogenic. It's true that tension can exacerbate pain—as when stress causes trigger points, which cause muscle tension. But tension is not the sole cause of RSI. This injury is not in your head; it's in your hands, wrists, arms, and shoulders! A doctor who refuses to look beyond his assumptions and insists that it's all in your head is selling you short.

If your doctor performs only a cursory exam without analyzing the potential causes of your injury and any aggravating factors, and then announces that it's all in your head, you have not been given adequate treatment. By educating yourself you can deal with people who are uninformed.

✄
DEALING WITH PAIN

Pain is a signal that your body has been or is being damaged. It may be acute (which occurs immediately after an injury), or it may be chronic (which is persistent and may last long after the initial injury). When you feel acute pain because of RSI, anything you do with your hands or arms will probably cause pain. Chronic pain may not afflict you around the clock, but it lasts longer. The special difficulty of chronic pain with RSI is that it should not be used as a reason to severely limit your activity. Once you are out of the acute-pain phase, carefully do what is necessary to restore strength and flexibility to your muscles, otherwise, you will continue to lose function. It takes getting to know your body to know what activities are acceptable and what limits are necessary to prevent further problems.

The pain of RSI can be overwhelming. People often use strong, vivid adjectives to describe their pain, words like *burning*, *throbbing*, and *flaming*, and phrases like *intense, shooting pain*, or *electrical currents*. Or it may not be so intense, but you find that your arms feel heavy or supersensitive. Even if you think it's bearable, it's not acceptable to be in pain. You're only doing damage to your body if you continue doing the activity that hurt you in the first place.

Pain, especially chronic, is difficult to deal with because its effects go far beyond the physical. Anyone suffering from the pain of RSI is likely to feel myriad conflicting emotions directly related to their pain. It's hard enough to cope with the physical pain but you also have to deal with other issues it caused, including uncertainty, isolation, expectations you or others may have about it, and fatigue. The following section details those issues. (Emotions will be discussed in more detail in chapter 11.)

Uncertainty

One of the hardest things to handle with RSI is not knowing if and when the pain will end. There's a fair amount of fear and anxiety that understandably goes along with that uncertainty. No scientific studies will indicate how long your injury is likely to last. If you have been dealing with your pain for a long time—and longer than a few days is a long time—it may seem as if it will last forever. But it won't, and it's important not to lose sight of that. It's so important to retain hope. Researchers have found that hope is one of the key components in successfully dealing with chronic pain.

Most physicians who treat RSI say that careful treatment and management can bring the pain under control. Yet the patient is frustrated because the road to recovery is never smooth. You may be feeling fine one day and then unwittingly do something that sets you back for days. Over time, you will get to know your body better and be able to avoid the peaks and valleys so common when you first begin treatment.

One way to keep yourself going is to seek support from others with RSI. Although each person's experience is unique, other sufferers often have valuable tips and insights to share. However, remember that a treatment that worked for one person may not be appropriate for another. But a support group can be a great way to get new ideas. More importantly, talking to someone who has dealt with it successfully over time can demonstrate that there *is* light at the end of the tunnel.

Isolation

Many books have been written about pain, and while the writers are often doctors who have treated patients with chronic pain, they rarely talk about experiencing the pain themselves. Anyone who *has* lived with the pain of RSI knows the frustration and isolation that come with it. Living with pain can be like living in a bubble, where you can see, hear, and talk to other people, but they can't really see or understand what you're experiencing. And most of the time, they don't really want to. For to acknowledge your pain means acknowledging the frightening thought that the same thing could happen to them.

Pain is also isolating for practical reasons: Your injury may prevent you from traveling comfortably, forcing you to stay at home more. RSI makes it hard to accomplish simple tasks, such as opening a door, so you'll probably find yourself limiting what you do in order to avoid causing yourself more pain. Coping with pain means stripping down your day so that you have fewer chores and responsibilities, which can mean more isolation.

Finally, pain is isolating because it's hard to talk about it. Nobody else cares about your pain in the same way that you do. Other people who are not in pain don't really want to talk about it because they don't know what to say or they're afraid they'll say the wrong thing. Sometimes, they will, and you'll be infuriated. The most offhand comment may make you seethe for days. Any anger you feel is probably justified but it won't help ease the isolation you feel.

One way to fight isolation is, again, to seek out support from others. (Support groups will be discussed in more detail in chapter 11.)

Expectations

Your own expectations will strongly influence how you deal with pain. You may not even be aware of your expectations, but they'll become obvious as you try to cope. If you feel you should have known better and not been injured in the first place, you'll wind up blaming yourself, which is self-defeating. Or, if you feel guilty about not being able to meet all your responsibilities at work or home, you may push yourself too hard and reinjure yourself. Conversely, if you feel others should take care of you because the injury wasn't your fault, you will spend more time and energy directed at getting them to do what you want rather than at your own care.

The expectations of others can make coping difficult as well. They may not understand why you are so debilitated and probably will expect you to bounce back much faster than is realistic. When you can't do that, they may feel disappointed and think that you have somehow failed. It's hard not to be hurt by such an attitude, especially since you may be feeling like a failure yourself. But it's not fair to blame the victim.

There may be other people who simply don't believe you're injured, but think you're faking it to get out of responsibilities at home or work. There's not much you can do about those insensitive types. But do be prepared if one of them gets RSI; you'll be the first one they'll turn to for advice!

Fatigue

It takes a lot of energy to deal with chronic pain. Simple tasks become a major challenge, and you have to figure out new ways to do them. Several seriously injured women used to joke about the fact that if they wanted to use the bathroom at work, they would wait until an able-bodied person got up to go through the door so that they could slip in behind them. Otherwise, opening the door would have been impossible.

Be on guard to avoid doing anything that will cause you more pain. Unfortunately, just what causes you problems is learned through painful trial and error. The more pain you feel, the more fatigue you feel.

Simply put, chronic pain is exhausting—and depressing. Allow yourself to slow down, and accept help from others when it is offered. It's hard to slow down, particularly for people who are used to working hard and being responsible. But the pain won't let up unless you do. That's not to say you should give up doing everything, because muscles actually heal better when they can move and remain pliable. But you need to adjust to a different, slower pace for a while.

Everyone handles pain differently. One person may be stoic, another hysterical. Neither coping mechanism is particularly useful in dealing with RSI. Being stoic may make it easier to deal with the people around you because most of them would rather not hear about your pain, but it will only create more opportunities to injure yourself further. There are times when you need to talk about your pain in order to get a change you need at work, for example, or a treatment recommended by your doctor. Being hysterical may garner immediate attention and sympathy for your injury, but it won't mean much support in the long term. And it may well inhibit you from doing what you need to do to get better.

There's no right way to react to intense, persistent pain, but you do need to find a way to cope that's useful for you.

�֍
YOUR GENERAL HEALTH

It's not uncommon for people diagnosed with RSI to take stock of their general health. It can't hurt to try to take better care of yourself through better nutrition, and getting more rest and exercise.

Paying attention to what you eat not only makes you feel better, but it makes your body more resilient. If you lack certain vital nutrients, that can contribute to health problems.

Some studies, for example, have found that a deficiency in the vitamin B_6 may be linked to carpal tunnel syndrome. Although that has been debated in the literature, the possibility is strong enough for some doctors to suggest that their carpal tunnel syndrome patients take up to 100 mg of B_6 a day. B_6 is considered relatively safe because it is a water-soluble vitamin, meaning it is flushed through your system fairly quickly; but it is still wise to avoid taking too much of it because excessive amounts might result in nerve damage.

Rather than trying to treat your RSI with specific vitamins, however, it's a better idea to try to eat regular meals made from fresh, whole foods. A high-salt diet can lead to water retention, which can exacerbate a condition such as carpal tunnel syndrome because it involves nerve compression. It's probably a good idea to limit or avoid caffeine, which is a central nervous system stimulant that causes constriction of the blood vessels. It may also contribute to stress, irritability, restlessness, and sleeplessness if consumed in excess. (Caffeine is found in coffee, tea, and colas, as well as in some medications, like aspirin. Take the time to read labels!)

Getting enough rest will also help you feel better. Study after study have shown that Americans simply don't get enough sleep. Researchers have warned about the dangers of trying to operate on a sleep deficit. Bear in mind that RSI is an *overuse* injury; part of getting yourself back on track is allowing your body to rest. If you are having trouble sleeping because of the pain or because you feel depressed, talk to your doctor. She may prescribe a low dosage of a medication temporarily to help you sleep.

Getting more rest may be a matter of letting yourself sit down and relax for a few minutes rather than trying to constantly accomplish something. People with RSI tend to be overachievers. It can be a big adjustment to have to slow down and take a break. But if you want to get better, take the time for yourself. Consider it part of your treatment.

Finally, exercise—once you no longer have acute pain— can be a potent tool in your recovery. It helps stimulate the production of endorphins, the body's natural painkillers, and reconditions your body. In short, it can help you heal and make you feel better at the same time. (Exercise will be discussed more thoroughly in the next chapter.)

The general rule of thumb in making changes to improve your health is moderation. It's not necessary to change your diet or routine completely in order to feel better. Small changes can make a big difference.

❧
STOPPING THE PAIN

A range of modalities, including medication and massage designed to stop your pain and speed your recovery, will be discussed in the next chapter. However, one of the most important things to remember is that if you find that a particular activity causes pain, stop doing it! If it's something that must be done, get help or find a way to do it that won't hurt. There's no reward for hurting yourself. A general rule of thumb is to use caution.

CHAPTER 8

WHAT YOU CAN EXPECT
IN TREATMENT

❈

*Stephanie Barnes, who directs the California-based
Association for Repetitive Motion Syndromes, fields
many calls from people all over the country with RSI.
Most, she says, want an answer to one question:
"What is the one thing I need to do to get better?"*

❈
NO MAGIC BULLET

Unfortunately, there is no one answer. Getting better takes
time and work. For some, it can become a second job; the
point is that recovery is a lot of work. Bear in mind, however,
that while recovery takes time, it will not take forever.

It is easy to become angry and discouraged. But, as with
any chronic injury, patience and perseverance will pay off.

The range of treatment options can be bewildering. Although no one model is recommended for all forms of RSI,

some common treatment modalities are typically used. They are designed to stop the pain and help you restore your strength and mobility, and most are conservative. They include rest, heat and cold, massage, electrical stimulation, medication, and exercise. A final option is surgery. None of the modalities discussed in this chapter should be done without a doctor's supervision.

❀
REST

This is a simple concept—the less you use your injured arms and hands, the less they'll hurt. It's easier said than done, however. Rest does not mean you should take to bed and do nothing (though there are some days when the pain may be so bad that that's all you'll want to do). Rest means setting aside unnecessary chores and responsibilities and not doing anything that will exacerbate your injury. It's not worth it to push to finish a project and deal with the pain later. The pain will only grow worse.

Rest also means getting enough sleep. Deep sleep is often interrupted by pain. Physical therapist Jackie Ross who has treated many cases of RSI, says 70 percent of her patients say they don't feel rested after a night's sleep. Yet rest, she maintains, is essential to give the muscles a chance to heal.

Splints

One frequently recommended treatment aimed at resting injured arms and hands is the use of splints. This is risky. Splints should be used only in a limited way and under a doctor's supervision. Never splint yourself.

Splints can alleviate pain because they immobilize hands and arms. If you can't move them, they won't hurt. But the danger is that muscles atrophy quickly. You can lose 20 percent of your tendon power and muscle strength within two weeks! The more strength you lose, the less you will be able to do. A phenomenon called progressive deconditioning, where you are able to do less and less, can occur. Just as conditioning exercises can make you steadily stronger, the lack of conditioning or using your muscles can cause progressive weakening. One woman remembers the terrifying day she couldn't muster the strength to turn the handle on a can opener. She immediately began a strengthening program and was able to regain her strength.

Scar tissue forms as your muscle and tendon tears heal, and the constant wearing of splints encourages that scar tissue to form in abnormal patterns because no movement is permitted by the splints. That can lead to a chronic injury.

The other problem splints pose is that they force you to use other muscles to compensate for those that are immobilized. Those muscles were not designed for the jobs normally done by the hands and arms, and as a result pain often will develop in those areas.

Different types of splints can help specific conditions, such as carpal tunnel syndrome or De Quervain's disease. A neutral wrist splint may be appropriate for carpal tunnel syndrome, and a thumb splint may be warranted for De Quervain's disease. In general, splints are particularly helpful for sleeping. Most people curl their hands and arms into positions they are not even aware of; those positions can exacerbate a condition like carpal tunnel syndrome. Sleeping with splints can help ease the symptoms. A splint being used for De Quervain's should prevent you from moving your thumb.

A variety of over-the-counter splints is sold. However, if you decide to get one, show it to your doctor before you wear it. He may recommend custom-designed splints instead. They should only be used as a treatment recommended by a doctor and not as a preventive measure. Some splint manufacturers claim in their advertisements that wearing splints can prevent carpal tunnel syndrome and other RSIs. A recent study by the University of California, San Francisco, found that people trying to prevent carpal tunnel syndrome should not wear splints. The researchers urged the federal government to take a closer look at manufacturers' ad claims.

To summarize, splints can be helpful when used judiciously to treat injuries specifically diagnosed by a doctor. Otherwise, don't use them. If you're already wearing one, try to wean yourself off it by wearing it for two hours and then taking it off for an hour. Fairly quickly, you'll be able to get rid of it.

Time Off

Your pain and injury may be so severe that you need to take some time off from work. This is always a difficult step. Even if your employer is sympathetic, you may be worried about job security or the resentment of your coworkers. Those are real concerns, but your priority must be your health.

In some cases, you may not be able to take time off, either because you cannot afford the loss in pay that usually goes along with any prolonged period out of work or you know you will lose your job. If either circumstance is the case, you may be entitled to ask for a temporary change of assignment or restricted duty so that you can take a break from the injurious activity. (More on your rights at work will be discussed in chapters 12 and 13.) If you are self-employed, such an option probably isn't available. One woman who was unable to continue her own business actually got a part-time job supervising a publishing project. She was able to earn temporary income while she focused most of her energy on physical therapy and recovery.

A knowledgeable doctor will try to strike the ideal balance between time off work and your return to work. To achieve that balance, good communication between the doctor, patient, and employer is essential.

✁
HEAT AND COLD

When you are in pain, you tend to tense your muscles, which leads to spasm; this leads to more pain. Heat and cold are used to reduce the spasm and stop this vicious cycle.

Heat

Heat increases blood flow to tendons, muscles, and ligaments near the skin's surface. Because good blood flow increases the supply of oxygen and nutrients, it promotes healing. If you are in the acute stage of injury, heat is not recommended immediately because it could exacerbate your inflammation. Heat doesn't ease swelling, painful scar tissue, or nerve damage either, but it can be useful in the treatment of chronic pain of RSI. Moist heat for muscles is generally better in promoting relaxation.

Heat treatment comes in a variety of forms—hot packs, hot towels, heat lamps, and warm baths. If you decide to use this form of treatment, it's best to follow the advice of your doctor or physical therapist.

Cold

Cold treatment is often recommended for sports injuries because it promotes constriction of blood circulation and numbs pain. It does the same for RSI and can be effective in reducing pain quickly.

Cold treatment also comes in a variety of forms—ice massage, ice packs, and ice baths. Or you can keep ice packs in the freezer and do the same thing yourself. It's easy to do at home or work. You can fill a paper cup with water and stick it in the freezer. To use it, simply take it out of the freezer and do the same thing. An ice bath is simply immersing your hands and arms in ice-cold water.

A general rule of thumb on using heat and cold: Use heat before activity in order to promote flexibility and relaxation, and use ice immediately after activity.

One caution: Cold packs are not appropriate for everyone. If you have a condition such as rheumatoid arthritis or diabetes, which makes you more susceptible to the cold, talk to your doctor before trying cold treatment.

Ultrasound

Ultrasound is one way to get heat to the deep tissues that superficial methods such as hot packs or massage cannot reach. With ultrasound, your therapist typically places gel on the injured area and then stimulates it with an ultrasound device, which uses high-frequency sound waves to generate heat in the injured area. Ultrasound helps to reduce pain and make scar tissue more elastic.

Paraffin bath

A paraffin bath is a heated metal container filled with melted paraffin, or wax, and wintergreen oil. It is used to get deep heat to the muscles and tendons of the hands. After dipping your hand several times to coat it with the hot paraffin, wrap it with plastic and cover it with a towel; allow it to cool. Then peel away the wax and gently stretch your hand.

Contrast Bath

Some doctors and physical therapists recommend combining heat with cold therapy. One method is the contrast bath, in which the patient immerses her hands and arms in warm to hot water for four minutes, then in cold water for one minute. The procedure is repeated up to four times for a total of twenty minutes. The set time periods for immersion in hot and cold water may vary; it's best to follow your doctor or therapist's instructions. Contrast baths reduce swelling, promote blood flow, and ease pain. They can be done several times a day.

✄
MASSAGE

Deep-tissue massage done by a skilled practitioner can be an invaluable part of your treatment. It promotes blood flow, which helps flush toxins out of muscles and tissues. It also helps ease painful muscle spasms by lengthening the muscle, and relaxes trigger points. It can help slow muscle atrophy. And one study found that patients receiving massage actually produced fewer stress-related hormones than patients who did not receive massage.

Massage has a long history as one of the healing arts, dating back to Greek and Roman times and to the T'ang Dynasty in China. Until recent years, massage was mainly a privilege of the wealthy, but now more and more medical practitioners are encouraging its use.

A good massage may not always be relaxing. It may even be uncomfortable at times, even slightly painful, in order to get at the problem. Some patients say they have to rest after a good massage but feel much better the next day. However, massage should never cause intense pain. Generally, a session lasts about an hour. Typically, some type of oil is applied to the skin to facilitate stroking.

Many different strokes are used in massage. A few of the strokes you are likely to encounter in a massage session are effleurage, which is a light stroking that is good for reducing swelling and promoting blood flow; petrissage, which is a firm friction stroking; kneading, which is a rhythmic lifting and squeezing of the flesh that helps stretch the muscles; range of motion, which is passive exercise aimed at mobilizing joints; and brushing, a light fingertip stroke often done at the end of a massage to spread general sensations over the body.

Unfortunately, massage is not something you or an untrained friend can do. You need a trained massage therapist with knowledge of human anatomy. Even more importantly, you must trust this person. Massage is an intimate experience and can be beneficial—but only if you trust your therapist. To find a good massage therapist, get a referral from someone you trust.

There are many different types of massage, from Swedish to medical. A knowledgeable physician can recommend the specific type you need. Some insurance plans pay for massage; it's worth checking to see if your plan or worker's compensation does. Some insurance companies consider it an alternative treatment. In some states, such as California, a professional massage practitioner must earn a certificate from an approved school. That certificate qualifies the massage therapist's services for insurance reimbursement.

ELECTRICAL STIMULATORS

A type of electrical stimulator commonly used to relieve pain is a transcutaneous electrical nerve stimulator, or TENS, a small box worn in a pocket or on your waist. It transmits low-voltage electrical impulses through wires to electrodes that are taped to the injured area. The electrical impulse travels over large nerve fiber tracts, which then inhibit the small nerve fiber tracts from transmitting pain. You will likely feel a tingling sensation while wearing it.

The idea is that a sufficient amount of stimulation can shut down pain. This is based on a theory of pain called *gate control*, which surmises that certain bundles of nerves actually act as gateways to pain; they can either open or close the pain sensation. In addition to inhibiting pain, the tingling of a TENS unit is supposed to help distract you. It may also stimulate painkilling endorphins, although the research on that is inconclusive.

The advantage of TENS is that you can use it at home or work and control the intensity of the electrical stimulation, thus giving you control over your treatment. The disadvantage is that it is a piece of equipment you must strap on. Some people also experience skin irritation from the unit's electrode paste.

Once you get the hang of it, a TENS unit is fairly easy to use. It can be purchased through medical-supply stores and if it is prescribed by your doctor, often it is covered by worker's compensation and insurance plans. Generally, it is not possible to get a TENS unit without a prescription.

✄
DRUGS

Many people flinch when they are advised to take medication. Despite the recent advances in developing a variety of anti-inflammatory drugs, some people feel that taking drugs to ease their pain can lead to dependency, and they don't want it to so mask the pain that they wind up injuring themselves further. These are valid concerns, and any prescribed drug should be taken exactly as directed. But don't rule out something that can be a valuable component of your treatment.

A more pressing concern is the issue of side effects. All drugs have them, but they may not always be bad. Talk to your doctor about the drug's side effects and how you can reduce any negative ones. You may find that any side effects you experience are tolerable and worth the pain reduction the medication provides.

It should be pointed out that medication is not a long-term solution. It is merely an aid to help you get the pain under control so that you can begin the hard work of rehabilitation. Nor is it a simple matter of prescribing one drug for all RSI patients' pain. The choice of medication may vary according to your weight, age, allergies, and other health issues. Some of the pain medications used for RSI patients include nonsteroidal anti-inflammatory drugs, aspirin and acetaminophen, antidepressants, muscle relaxants, and steroids.

NSAIDs

Nonsteroidal anti-inflammatory drugs (NSAIDs) are often prescribed for the pain and swelling caused by RSI. One of the most common is ibuprofen (Advil, Nuprin, and Motrin).

Ibuprofen can be helpful, but in some people it also can cause side effects such as stomach irritation, constipation, or diarrhea. Some patients risk increased bleeding or drowsiness with this category of drug. Nonetheless, NSAIDs can be useful in treating pain caused by inflammation.

Nonsteroidal anti-inflammatory drugs are generally given in pill form. For most of them, it's advisable to take the pills on a full stomach to reduce the risk of stomach pain and nausea. Taking them at meals is also an easy way to remind yourself that it's time for your medication. The drugs vary in the number of times they must be taken daily. Ibuprofen must be taken three to four times a day to be helpful; Feldene, which has a longer blood-level time, is taken once a day. Because people respond differently to different drugs, you may have to try more than one before you get the necessary relief. There are no known long-term effects of taking nonsteroidal anti-inflammatory drugs.

Aspirin and Acetaminophen

Aspirin is an anti-inflammatory agent that can be as effective as other nonsteroidal anti-inflammatory drugs and is much cheaper. It should not be taken with any other nonsteroidal anti-inflammatory drugs. However, it can be taken with acetaminophen (Tylenol) for excellent pain relief. Aspirin seems to be more effective for acute pain than chronic pain. Acetaminophen does not reduce inflammation, but it can reduce pain. As with any medication, watch the dosage of acetaminophen. Because excessive use can cause liver damage, many doctors believe the dosage should be limited to 2,000 to 4,000 milligrams a day.

Antidepressants

You may balk at the idea of taking an antidepressant for your pain because you may think your doctor is implying that the pain is in your head. However, antidepressants have been found to relieve pain in patients who are not depressed. They have been used to treat headaches, premenstrual syndrome, panic attacks, fibromyalgia, and chronic fatigue syndrome. Although not well explained in the scientific literature, one possible explanation for their effectiveness is that people who develop chronic pain develop a serotonin imbalance and certain antidepressants help correct that imbalance. The pain relief, in effect, is a side effect of the antidepressant. When one is prescribed for pain relief, the dosage is usually lower than that used for treating depression. It should be noted that antidepressants are safe for most patients.

Two main types of antidepressants are used for treating pain—tricyclic antidepressants, which include Elavil, Pamelor, and Desyrel; and selective serotonin reuptake inhibitor antidepressants, which include Zoloft, Paxil, and Prozac. Tricyclic antidepressants are likely to be used first because most doctors have more experience with them, but both types are used for pain relief. Side effects of tricyclics include dry mouth, drowsiness, and dizziness when you first stand up. Side effects of selective serotonin reuptake inhibitors (SSRIs) include headaches, gastrointestinal distress, decreased appetite, insomnia or drowsiness, and sexual problems. Tricyclics can be harmful if taken with alcohol. Selective serotonin reuptake inhibitors are generally safe if taken with alcohol, but the combination can cause drowsiness.

It is not uncommon to feel depressed by the pain and disability RSI causes. Although depression will be discussed in more depth in chapter 10, it's worthwhile to point out here that depression exacerbates pain. It's difficult to diagnose this because your doctor may assume your pain is worse because your condition is worsening. If you have symptoms of depression, seek help specifically for it.

If your sleep is interrupted by your RSI symptoms, your doctor may recommend a medication. A small dose of an antidepressant can be helpful; it can aid in longer, more restful sleep, which is essential for healing. Without it, your recovery will be slowed considerably.

Muscle Relaxants

In some cases, a muscle relaxant, such as Valium, Flexeril, or Robaxin, may be prescribed. They don't act directly on the muscles; it is believed that they work by relaxing the entire central nervous system, which allows your muscles to relax. They can be particularly effective in treating muscle spasms. Muscle relaxants are particularly useful when stress is a strong contributing factor. However, they are not recommended for long-term use.

Rules for Taking Medication

Most of us have taken some kind of medication, so much so that it's easy to take it for granted. To be sure that the medication works properly and safely, take it seriously.

- *Ask questions.* Be an informed consumer. Ask your doctor how the medication is taken and if there are any side effects. If your doctor's answer doesn't satisfy you, ask your pharmacist. Most pharmacists love to be asked questions about specific drugs. If he has substituted a generic drug, ask what the difference is. Learn as much as you can about what to expect after you take the medication.

- *Follow instructions.* Pay attention to the warnings and instructions on taking the medication. There are reasons for these instructions. Follow them. If you don't, you cannot expect relief.
- *Give it time.* Bear in mind that it often takes time for a new medicine or increased dosage to have any effect. Sometimes it can take weeks or even months so you must allow some time before giving up. If you are not feeling any results, inform your doctor. You may need to change medications, or you may simply need to give it more time.
- *Be honest.* It's vital to tell your doctor about any other drugs you may be taking because of the potential interactions. Some drugs, like birth control pills, may have become such a habit that you forget you're taking them. Take time to think about what you're ingesting and tell your doctor. In addition, discuss any fears or concerns you have about medications.
- *Report any side effects.* If you experience side effects, tell your doctor immediately. Although concern about side effects is legitimate, they are not an issue for most people. With the exception of aspirin, fewer than one person in twenty has to stop taking a drug because of negative side effects. About one in six people is taken off aspirin because of the bad side effects.

Cortisone

Cortisone is somewhat controversial because it is such a strong medicine, but it has been found to be helpful when other modes of treatment have not worked. Cortisone is generally given by injection, in creams, or sprays. Injections are typically given by a doctor; the cortisone creams, typically containing about 10 percent cortisone, are administered by therapists who use it to reduce inflammation. It can also be taken in pill form, although this is not generally used for RSI, except in cases of reflex sympathetic disorder.

A cortisone injection can be tricky and should only be given by a skilled practitioner. Typically, a local anesthetic such as Novocain or lidocaine is given to numb the area. Then the injection is given, and pain relief should be felt almost immediately. A cortisone injection can be useful for treatment of an inflamed bursa, which may be irritated by other treatments. The cortisone can stop the pain and prevent the formation of scar tissue. It's effective because the medication is delivered directly to the inflamed area. In selected cases, it can be helpful for carpal tunnel syndrome.

EXERCISE

If you are in physical therapy for treatment of RSI, your therapist probably has you on a program of stretching and strengthening exercises. Research has shown that exercise—gradually introduced after an injury—helps you get back to normal faster. It helps to recondition your muscles, prevent reinjury, and relieve the stress of chronic pain.

If you have a busy life, it may be difficult to find time to exercise. Work, family, and other commitments can eat up spare time, but exercise doesn't have to be time-consuming. You may want to start out with fifteen minutes and gradually build up to half an hour. If you make it a part of your daily routine, exercise will become a habit. If you skip it, don't beat yourself up or give up. Even a little exercise is better than nothing.

However, you shouldn't exercise if you are in acute pain. Vigorous activity during the early acute phase can cause further injury; it makes more sense to rest. Once you are beyond the acute phase, you may still be unconsciously guarding yourself against pain—holding your muscles rigid, or hunching your shoulders inward in a protective position. That protective posture is no longer useful once you're out of acute pain. It is then that you should consider gentle exercise. Before doing anything, however, discuss it with your doctor.

Stretching

Stretching helps lengthen muscles that are shortened by spasm. That, in turn, allows more blood to reach the muscles, which promotes healing. Stretching also helps restore flexibility to muscles, which enables them to withstand greater shock, and reduces the tension that accumulates during strenuous activity.

Some physicians suggest doing computer stretches throughout the day. As mentioned previously, researchers have not found that such stretches prevent injury. But stretching is a good first step toward developing an exercise program and can help speed your recovery.

If you find it boring, consider a yoga class to keep you motivated. Yoga emphasizes awareness of breath and body movements. It has been shown to help condition the body slowly, increasing both flexibility and strength. A class is a good way to begin, although plenty of videos are available for beginners.

There are some important rules to remember about stretching:

- Don't bounce. Stretch slowly and gently.
- Hold your stretches for fifteen to twenty seconds.

- Stretch to the point of resistance, not pain.
- Try to breathe deeply and rhythmically with your stretches.
- Try to make them a part of your daily routine.

Strengthening

Any stretching program is likely to be accompanied by strengthening exercises. Anyone who has RSI knows how quickly muscle weakness and fatigue can set in. Strengthening exercises are a way to recondition your muscles so that they can return to a normal state.

Strengthening exercises vary. You may begin with simple isometric exercises and then build up to gentle resistance exercises, such as creating resistance by using a band. Gradually, you may start lifting weights—though for people seriously debilitated by RSI, the weights should be light. One RSI patient ruefully remembers starting out doing her exercises with 6-ounce cans of tomato paste because that was all the weight she could bear. She remembers how thrilled she was when she "graduated" to 12-ounce cans of soda.

If you lift weights, particularly in a gym, it is important to warm up and to cool down. General stretching beforehand does not constitute a warm-up; your warm-up should be geared toward the activity you will perform. A standard rule of thumb is to warm up the specific joints that will be used in the exercise.

When doing strengthening exercises, consider the following rules:

- Do your exercises slowly.
- Increase your weight gradually.
- Always do warm-up stretches before you begin.
- If you feel pain, stop.

• Try to breathe deeply and rhythmically as you do your exercises.
• Make them a part of your daily routine.

Aerobic Exercise

Low-impact aerobic exercise can be fun, speed healing, and make you feel better. This should be approached carefully, because even though you may think you feel better, you may not be ready to rush into a full-scale program. As with stretching and strengthening exercises, begin any aerobic exercise program gradually.

Swimming is often recommended as a reconditioning exercise because it permits you to stretch and strengthen your muscles while your body is weightless. That means your muscles do not have to absorb shock, as they do when you run, for instance. Using a stationary bicycle can be a good aerobic exercise, as long as you don't grip the handlebars too tightly. A treadmill provides a good workout as well.

With any exercise, don't do anything that causes your symptoms to flare up. The goal is to exercise to just below your pain threshold. And before doing anything, check with your doctor.

Though it may seem a nuisance in the beginning, exercise can yield big payoffs. One immediate benefit is that it helps stimulate your endorphins, which are the body's natural painkillers. Finally, exercise not only helps recondition your body but it also increases your body awareness—which will help you spot warning signals or prevent further pain or reinjury.

Even moderate exercise, like brisk walking, can be beneficial. Studies have shown that sedentary people can achieve significant gains from moderate exercise. It not only lowers heart attack risk, but it also lowers blood pressure, helps fight stress,

and strengthens the immune system. In bad weather, it's easy
to move your walk indoors. Some twenty-four hundred shopping malls let walkers in before shopping hours. There are
even walking clubs at many of these malls!

Exercise is an appealing option to some people with RSI
because it enables them to do something about their condition rather than passively wait for it to improve. In fact, most
of the conservative treatments discussed here require that the
patient be actively involved. When you are able to participate
in your recovery, it not only is more successful, it's more
enjoyable.

Many RSIs can be treated effectively with a range of conservative treatments. If you don't think your RSI is responding
to treatment as you had hoped, ask yourself if you are following
your treatment and rehabilitation plan, if you are being careful
not to do things that would cause reinjury, and if you are trying
to do too much too soon. Be honest. If you are doing everything
as your doctor and therapist have directed, and your injury is
still not responding, surgery may be a last resort.

SURGERY

Most physicians recommend surgery only if they feel that conservative treatments will not be effective in treating the injury.

Carpal tunnel surgery is one of the most commonly performed surgeries in the United States—some two hundred
thousand a year. It's relatively easy and often effective. Yet,
many doctors believe that it is overused. It's a difficult issue.
Because other conditions can mimic the symptoms of carpal
tunnel syndrome, there may be cases where a misdiagnosis led
to surgery. However, when carpal tunnel syndrome is accurately diagnosed, surgery can offer immediate relief. And some

doctors fear that the longer you put it off, the more the median nerve will be irritated. And the longer the nerve is irritated, the less likely successful surgery will be.

Nerve-conduction tests and/or the results of an electromyogram should be used to help make the decision to have surgery for carpal tunnel syndrome, but the most important issue is your quality of life. You need enough information to judge whether surgery will improve the quality of your life.

Good surgeons won't operate unless they think it's necessary. Before submitting to surgery, you should ask the following questions:

- Why is it necessary?
- Could I choose a more conservative course of treatment that won't risk more damage?
- Do I risk more damage if I don't have the surgery?
- What are the possible complications of surgery?
- What are the chances of the surgery doing what it is supposed to?
- How many times has my doctor performed this procedure?
- Are there any problems that could arise?
- Will it improve my life?

In making your decision, you'll have to weigh the pros and cons. It's helpful to get a second opinion. Even if your doctor tries to minimize your fears by telling you it's a minor procedure, any surgery is a major event in your life. It's a big deal because it's your body.

In carpal tunnel surgery, the transverse ligament is cut and released, which relieves the pressure on the median nerve. Recovery time varies, depending on the degree of damage to the median nerve and the technique used by the surgeon. Although carpal tunnel surgery has a high success rate, it can fail. The nerve may have been irreparably damaged prior to surgery, or the scar tissue from the surgery may actually put more pressure on the nerve.

Surgery is also sometimes recommended for De Quervain's disease or ulnar-nerve entrapment.

Miriam, who had surgery on both hands after being diagnosed with severe carpal tunnel syndrome, recalls having a difficult recovery from her second surgery, which was on the left hand. When the stitches were removed, she returned to her bookstore job, but within a few weeks, the pain in both hands was so great that she was given three weeks of disability leave and part-time work. Her right hand, on which the first surgery had been done, was in pain because she had overused it trying to compensate for her other hand. Although she wore splints and tried to be careful, she says, "It's really a difficult situation to have surgery on your hands—unless you're a princess."

She says she has a better understanding of her limits and tries to manage her RSI by using splints when she has to shelve books or carry them to another part of the store. She swims at least twice a week and does a lot of walking to try to keep in shape. When her hands flare up, she takes a paper cup that she has filled with water, and frozen, and rubs the ice over the painful areas. Whenever she gets a new manager at her store, she makes a point of explaining her limits. And when she wants to do something she knows might cause her pain, like tilling her garden, she enlists the help of a friend. "I take my hands very seriously," she says.

For Miriam, recovery has become a matter of managing her RSI. "I think doctors and physical therapists can give you advice," she says, "but you yourself have to learn to deal with it."

CHAPTER 9

ALTERNATIVE
THERAPIES

✤

*When John, a computer programmer in California,
was diagnosed with RSI in 1991, he initially tried
conventional treatment. He consulted a doctor, wore
splints, and saw a physical therapist. He followed his
therapist's instructions, but after a few months, John
showed no improvement and, in fact, seemed to be
getting worse. Finally, his therapist said to him,
"C'mon, John. You've got to get yourself better."*

*She was right. "I realized, yeah, it was up to me,"
he says.*

*That's when John's journey through alternative
therapies began. He saw a chiropractor, went to a
health clinic that specialized in massage and colonics
(a therapy in which the large intestine is irrigated),
and dramatically changed his diet. He weaned himself
from splints—"I decided that I had to stop looking*

ill"—*and started lifting weights. And he underwent a spiritual healing in which members of his spiritual group put him in a healing circle and prayed.*

It took John three years to restore his health. He is now back at work full time as a computer programmer. He says the journey has not stopped for him, that he is still learning, but, he says, "I am a different person now."

❀
SEEKING ALTERNATIVES

It is not uncommon for people with RSI to feel frustrated with standard medical treatment. Doctors don't have all the answers, recovery takes a long time, and it doesn't always progress smoothly. Anyone who has experienced chronic pain knows it is more than a physical experience; in fact, in the nineteenth century, physicians thought pain was an emotion. For some people, it makes sense to explore holistic healing arts that emphasize the mind-body connection. Or as one man with a severe case of RSI put it, "When you've been in this kind of pain for months, you'll try anything!"

If you decide to try an alternative therapy, *tell your doctor.* One comprehensive medical survey found that more than two-thirds of patients of all types who had tried an alternative therapy did not tell their doctor. It's not always easy to tell your doctor, especially if she is skeptical of holistic medicine. However, it's your responsibility as a patient to keep your doctor informed. An experienced and understanding physician will rarely object if she feels the therapy won't do you any harm. Some of the therapies discussed in this chapter are used widely enough in hospitals and clinics that they probably shouldn't be labeled *alternative.* In fact, some insurance companies reimburse for certain alternative or holistic therapies.

One warning: If you decide to try an alternative therapy, keep it in perspective. Don't use it as an excuse to avoid what's going on with your body. It can be a useful adjunct to your therapy, but it's not a substitute. And don't use it as a means of self-diagnosis; as always, diagnosis should be left to your doctor.

The therapies in this chapter include relaxation techniques, energy balance therapies, chiropractic, osteopathy, homeopathy, various methods of body work, magnetic therapy, and nutritional therapy. The brief descriptions that follow are not intended to be an endorsement of a particular therapy but should provide some guidance to those interested in exploring an alternative therapy for treatment of RSI.

❊
RELAXATION TECHNIQUES

Relaxation techniques have become fairly commonplace in hospitals and clinics as a means of reducing stress, which can contribute to muscle tension and pain. Specialists in the field point out that our bodies unconsciously react physically to many situations as though they were life threatening—the fight or flight response. That response, which includes tensed muscles, constricted blood vessels, and increased heart and blood rates, is appropriate when the situation is life-threatening. Typically, however, it is not, and many researchers believe the response contributes to stress-related ailments. Relaxation techniques are a way to minimize and control that response.

Research also has confirmed the efficacy of relaxation techniques in promoting healing. The benefits for lowering blood pressure and anxiety levels have been well documented. Among the techniques to be discussed here are visualization, meditation, biofeedback, and flotation therapy.

Visualization

Visualization, or guided imagery, is a technique used in hypnosis. It is fairly simple. You close your eyes, breathe deeply, and imagine a restful, pleasant place where you would like to be. When beginning, the image arises gradually, as you imagine yourself going there. As you become more practiced, you will be able to summon the image more quickly. It becomes a way of taking a refreshing break. If you are in pain, it can make your pain more tolerable or distract you from it altogether.

Visualization is also used as a healing technique. Some hypnotherapists help patients come up with images aimed at promoting healing. You might, for example, imagine blood flowing to your arms and hands, bringing nutrients to the areas that need them most. Or, if your arms and hands feel tight, you might imagine bands falling away. Audiotapes can help you do such visualizations on your own, or you could try consulting a hypnotherapist.

Visualization has had documented effects on eliminating and/or reducing pain. People who have used visualization rather than anesthetic have reported that the pain of surgery was numbed. As with any discipline, if you want to see results, you've got to practice, practice, practice.

Meditation

Meditation is similar to the relaxed state achieved through visualization. The practice is central to many religions, but it has also become a well-known and widely used relaxation technique. To do it, sit in a comfortable posture and strive to empty your mind of thoughts by focusing on a particular object or sound. With smooth, regular breathing, you can achieve a state of relaxation.

Research has shown that meditation can slow heart rate and respiration, thereby reducing stress. Regular practitioners of meditation report decreased anxiety, depression and tension, and increased concentration and resilience. It is best learned from a teacher, but many books and audiotapes are available if you want to do it on your own.

Biofeedback

Biofeedback is a type of relaxation therapy in which you are hooked up to a machine—usually by electrodes—that monitors heart rate, body temperature, and muscle tension. The machine itself does not cause you to relax. Instead, by giving you visual or auditory cues, it helps you control your body's reactions. The visual cues might be a line spiking on a graph on a computer monitor; the auditory cues might be a beep that becomes more frequent as your muscles tense. With training, biofeedback helps you recognize when you are experiencing tension that may lead to pain, and then find a way to relax to avoid its onset.

Researchers aren't sure what mechanism makes biofeedback work, but they have documented its medical benefits. It may be due to the constant feedback that enables you to make physiological changes—either consciously or unconsciously—or it may be due to the sense of self-control over your symptoms. Or it may be due to both. It is clear, however, that people have more control over involuntary bodily functions than was previously thought.

Biofeedback is used in hospitals, clinics, or a private practitioner's office. A trainer teaches exercises that help you relax. Training may take weeks or months, but generally lasts six to ten weeks. Some insurance companies will pay for it.

A responsible biofeedback therapist will not treat you

until you have had a thorough physical exam. Find a biofeedback therapist by asking your doctor for a referral, or call the psychology or psychiatry departments at a local university. In addition, local medical or biofeedback societies may be of help. The Biofeedback Certification Institute of America, based in Wheat Ridge, Colorado, publishes a directory of practitioners. (For a phone number, see the appendix.)

Flotation Therapy

In flotation therapy, a tank is filled with highly salted, room temperature water. The level of Epsom salts is so high that it supports the body, making floating effortless. The tank is usually enclosed with a switch to turn on a light, although there are some open flotation tanks. The idea is to place you in a comfortable environment with restricted light and sound, which enables you to relax. Flotation therapists say the tank does two things: It refocuses attention on internal stimuli, and it rebalances the body. The combination of relaxation, weightlessness, and Epsom salts is believed to relieve pain, in part by stimulating the production of endorphins.

Flotation tanks are used in some clinics to treat people with chronic pain. They are also used to help patients reduce anxiety, as well as treat addictive behaviors, such as cigarette smoking. Some research has shown flotation tanks to be effective in modifying smoking behavior.

❧

ENERGY BALANCE THERAPIES

Energy balance therapies focus on the idea that each person has an energy field. Using different approaches, each of these therapies seeks to balance that field because practitioners believe that a balanced energy field helps to restore a person to health. It's a relativistic approach to treatment of health problems rather than seeking a particular cause and effect. The idea that each person has an aura or subtle energy field is not new. Stories of healers have been told in almost all religions throughout the world.

Acupuncture

A centuries-old Chinese healing art, acupuncture is based on the flow of energy throughout the body. Acupuncturists believe the body is divided into energy *meridians*. When such a meridian is blocked, pain and weakness can result. Using tiny, sterilized needles, an acupuncturist gently stimulates a precise point or points along the body's meridians. The needle may be twisted or coupled with a weak electrical current to stimulate the area. The point at which a needle is inserted may be far removed from the area of pain, but it is done to stimulate a healthy energy flow.

Acupuncture is used to relieve specific symptoms and promote general well-being, and researchers have found that it stimulates the production of endorphins. Although theories of why it works vary, acupuncture has become fairly well accepted among Western medical practitioners. One recent study published in Great Britain found that patients with chronic epicondylitis (tennis elbow) had significant pain relief after just one acupuncture treatment.

If you decide to try an acupuncturist, choose someone who uses sterilized, disposable needles. Many states license acupuncturists, and it is preferable, of course, to find someone who is licensed. Some insurance companies will reimburse you for acupuncture treatment, even through the worker's compensation system. You can try to find a physician who is also an acupuncturist by calling the referral service of the

American Academy of Medical Acupuncture. (Check the appendix for the phone number.)

Acupressure

Acupressure is another Chinese healing art based on the concept of energy meridians, but it uses fingertip pressure rather than needles to balance energy flow and relieve ailments. The pressure can help to relieve trigger point pain by diffusing built-up lactic acid.

Acupressure also has become a generic term for the various strokes used by some massage therapists and physical therapists. As in acupuncture, pressure on one part of the body can relieve pain in a different part of the body. This is not such a radical idea when you understand the theory of referred pain, in which pain from an injury may actually be felt in a different spot in the body.

Acupressure is generally regarded as safe. In addition, it is easy to teach so that you can use it yourself when needed.

Therapeutic Touch

Therapeutic touch, developed by a New York University nursing professor named Dolores Krieger, is based on the ancient concept of the healing power of the laying on of hands. Typically, the practitioner of therapeutic touch does not actually touch the patient. Instead, the practitioner, placing her hands two to four inches above the body, smoothes out or shifts the energy field that surrounds the human body.

Research has found that patients treated with therapeutic touch experience certain physiological changes, such as decreased anxiety and increased relaxation. This is important because anxiety and pain are intertwined. A New York University study found that postoperative patients treated with therapeutic touch did not report an actual reduction in pain but were able to go longer periods before needing pain medication. Another study of ninety hospitalized cardiovascular patients found that the group receiving therapeutic touch showed a significantly greater reduction in anxiety than the groups that did not receive it.

Before a session, the practitioner of therapeutic touch typically meditates briefly to become centered on the healing. One study found that nurses who did not do this before a session had no significant effect on their patients. That focus apparently helps empower the practitioner, or healer, who can then discern imbalances in the patient's energy field. The ability of a practitioner to know where you are experiencing pain can be extraordinary. A session usually does not last longer than thirty minutes.

Currently, there is no certification for therapeutic touch because it began as a modality for nurses who have medical training.

CHIROPRACTIC

Chiropractors use a series of manipulative techniques to treat neuromuscular problems. They focus on the spine, believing that good alignment is essential to good health. They believe adjusting the spine can help ease or eliminate symptoms. They also tend to concentrate on localized problem areas rather than general stretching and massage, although some chiropractors offer those modalities as part of their treatment.

Chiropractors are traditionally associated with treating back problems, but today, most treat a range of physical problems, from carpal tunnel syndrome to migraines. Many people associate "back cracking" with chiropractors, but, in fact, the adjustments are more subtle, varied, and sophisticated. Although more traditional chiropractors do limit themselves to adjusting the spine, many use other treatment modalities, such as ultrasound, to supplement their treatment.

The term *subluxation* is used by chiropractors to describe defective joint movement. Your chiropractor will determine whether you have a subluxation through the combination of a physical exam and X rays, and then try to mobilize the area to realign it. He may also examine your posture and suggest lifestyle or work changes to ease your symptoms.

Although the American Medical Association labeled chiropractic as "an unscientific cult" as recently as 1963, chiropractic appears to have won growing acceptance in the traditional medical community. Some hospitals grant licensed chiropractors access to their facilities for a limited range of services, and the AMA now allows its members to associate with any legally sanctioned medical professional. In addition, many insurers will pay for chiropractic treatment.

Because the treatment is so physical, take care in choosing a chiropractor. As with any medical treatment, be an informed consumer.

OSTEOPATHY

Osteopaths are trained medical doctors who use a range of manipulative techniques to relieve pain, restore mobility, and promote general well-being. Osteopaths place particular emphasis on the musculoskeletal system, which comprises two-thirds of the body's mass. Like chiropractors, osteopaths believe the alignment of the body is vital. Unlike chiropractors, osteopaths can prescribe drugs to treat an illness. They also can specialize in all areas of medicine, from neurosurgery to psychiatry.

Osteopathic medicine emphasizes the interrelationship of structure and function. Osteopaths believe all of the body's systems work together. In treatment, the osteopath is likely to pay attention not only to the problem area but also to other parts of the body that may be contributing to the problem. The focus is on the whole body, as a unit. One defective part can influence the entire body. The best conditions for recovery are to treat not only the injured area but to provide optimum conditions for the entire body.

In an exam, an osteopath asks a number of questions about your general health and lifestyle, assesses posture and balance, and checks the ease of movement of various body parts. Like any other medical doctor, the osteopath is likely to use palpation and simple observation to help make the diagnosis. Once the structural exam is completed, the osteopath will perform a physical exam and review your medical history to determine a treatment plan.

Osteopaths have an appreciation for the body's ability to heal itself. They are concerned with the maintenance of health, as well as the cure. Part of treatment is to educate you about good health and the avoidance of disease or injury; osteopaths recognize, however, that medication and/or surgery may be necessary elements of treatment.

HOMEOPATHY

The basic premise of homeopathy is simply that like cures like. Homeopaths believe the same substance that causes an illness, when administered in highly diluted doses, can also cure it. The medicines a homeopath uses are called *tinctures*, which are highly diluted and shaken extracts of natural ingredients. Typically, a homeopath chooses a single remedy for treatment.

Homeopaths believe symptoms are *signs* of a problem. A fever, for example, is not really the problem but a symptom of a problem and is, in fact, one mechanism the body uses to fight infection. Rather than treating the symptom, homeopaths seek to treat the underlying problem. With that in mind, a homeopath is likely to ask you questions to determine your temperament and life-style, as well as your physical condition.

Many advocates of homeopathy believe it is good for treating chronic problems. When someone is cured, homeopaths believe a standard pattern has been followed: A remedy works from the top of the body downward, from the inside out, and symptoms clear in reverse order of their appearance. Homeopaths say it is particularly good for treating musculoskeletal injuries such as RSI because it reduces swelling, helps to relieve pain, and promotes tissue healing.

Homeopathic medicine is recognized by the U.S. Food and Drug Administration as drugs, but are typically cheaper than conventional medicine, costing an average of three dollars to seven dollars a bottle.

Although homeopathy is not covered by U.S. insurance companies, it is fully reimbursable under the French social security system, the German national health system, and the British national health service.

BODY WORK

Because posture can play such an important role in developing RSI, body work techniques are often recommended to people with RSI as a way of improving posture. Among them are the Alexander technique, Feldenkrais, yoga, myotherapy, t'ai chi ch'uan, and Rolfing.

Alexander Technique

Probably the most famous story about the Alexander technique is one about its founder, F. Matthias Alexander. An actor, he developed a chronic hoarseness. Studying his posture in a mirror, he noticed that even while he was preparing to speak he would pull back his head and tighten his throat. Over time, he developed ways of holding his neck, head, and body that reduced the stress on his throat. Oddly, his normal posture felt comfortable, while his new, healthier posture felt strange. He stuck to it, however, and his hoarseness never returned. At the same time, his voice became clearer, and he developed greater stage presence.

That was the genesis of the Alexander technique, which is a way to retrain the body to eliminate unhealthy postures. Its underlying theory is that the body loses its natural, healthy posture in response to stresses. As Alexander began to observe others, he noticed that he was not alone in having developed bad posture and inhibited movements. He saw a need for teaching others, and his clientele quickly spread beyond actors to scientists and physicians.

The Alexander technique takes time and practice, under the guidance of a trained instructor, because bad postural habits are difficult to change. The method's focus is the positioning of the head so that it can be properly balanced while the neck muscles are relaxed. An instructor will teach you how to do something as simple as sit in a chair and stand up again. At first, the new method of sitting may feel awkward, but eventually, people using the Alexander technique often say they feel lighter and healthier.

The group keeps a list of certified members. The key to the success of the Alexander technique is practice. You must be motivated to learn and stick with it, but Alexander teachers say the payoff is worth the investment. (For more information on the technique and how to find a teacher, see the appendix.)

Feldenkrais

The primary goal of Feldenkrais is to teach you body awareness through movement. The idea is that the healing is promoted by greater awareness of the body. Feldenkrais's founder, an Israeli physicist named Moshe Feldenkrais, believed that each repeated movement sends a signal to the brain and, in effect, lays down a pattern that is subsequently followed. The Feldenkrais method is designed to break such patterns and teach students how to change distorted posture and movement.

Typically, Feldenkrais is taught in a group session. The teacher takes the class through a series of movements in which students are expected to focus on the part of the body being moved and the sensations associated with it. Students are not only taught how to move but also learn how to release muscle tension. Usually, lessons begin with a simple movement, like flexing your foot, and progress to more complex movements, like sitting and standing. The exercises are deceptively simple, yet they can teach a great deal about your body. (For more information about Feldenkrais, see the appendix.)

Yoga

Although yoga developed literally centuries ago as a spiritual discipline, it is often taught in the West as a primarily physical exercise. Many consider it a good rehabilitative tool because it combines gentle stretching with a low-impact workout. There are many different types of yoga, with varying levels of activity. Though all yoga styles emphasize stretching and breathing, some provide a fairly strenuous workout. Other styles emphasize meditation. It is up to you to choose the style that suits you; you may have to try several before you find a good fit.

As with any discipline, it's easier to keep it up if you take a class. If you prefer to try it on your own, there are many videotapes available with yoga exercises. (However, it is a good idea to start out with some training from a knowledgeable teacher because some yoga poses, if done incorrectly or held too long, can cause muscle strains or other injuries.)

Medical researchers have found that yoga has a wide array of benefits, from general conditioning and stress reduction to improved functioning of the heart and lungs. Yoga devotees who use it for more than physical exercise say it is a way to achieve spiritual harmony and the union of mind, body, and soul.

Myotherapy

Myotherapy is a technique aimed at diffusing trigger points, which are tight and often knotted spots in the muscles that can be tender or painful. Developed by fitness expert Bonnie Prudden, it consists of a series of manual techniques in which firm, sustained pressure is applied to release the trigger points. The goal of myotherapy is to provide more than a temporary fix; it seeks to eliminate the trigger point and re-educate the muscles—through gentle stretching and exercise—to prevent it from developing again.

T'ai Chi Ch'uan

Also known as t'ai chi, this ancient Chinese system of moving meditation is also a martial art. In it, students practice gentle, flowing movements in precise patterns that can last from five minutes to half an hour, the average being about ten minutes.

Although the patterns, called *forms* by teachers, look effortless, they require considerable coordination and mental focus. Emphasis is placed on precision of movement, as well as breathing.

One particular benefit of t'ai chi for people with RSI is its emphasis on posture. Achieving near-ideal posture is one of the practice's fundamental goals. The basic stance, in which the knees are bent slightly, causes a small bend in the back and minimizes the curvature of the neck and back. The attention to alignment helps relax the body so that it assumes the proper posture naturally.

The practice of t'ai chi is designed to balance your *chi*, or life force. Practitioners say it helps develop balance, achieve control, and relieve stress. Although there has not been much significant research into the area of t'ai chi and stress, one Australian study found that t'ai chi was as effective as meditation and brisk walking in reducing levels of some stress hormones in men and women. Other anecdotal evidence points to t'ai chi's beneficial effects on insomnia and high blood pressure. Some people report experiencing a meditative state when they do a form.

Although the movements of t'ai chi are gentle and flowing, they can also be powerful tools for self-defense. T'ai chi is often recommended for people who want an exercise that will not force or strain their muscles.

Books and videos about t'ai chi are available, but a class is probably the best way to learn it because of its subtle points of form and posture. When choosing a class, ask about its emphasis. Some classes focus on the self-defense aspect of the art, while others stress the fitness aspect of it.

Rolfing

Like many other alternative therapies, Rolfing is designed to restore balance to the human body, with the idea that healing comes from balance. Basically, Rolfing consists of ten sessions of deep, manipulative techniques aimed at increasing muscle length and aligning the body. Named after its founder, Ida Rolf, it has a reputation for being painful. In some cases, it is, though Rolfers say it isn't nearly as painful as people think.

Rolfing became connected with the human potential movement in the 1970s because Ida Rolf treated Fritz Perls, the founder of Gestalt therapy, at his Esalen Institute. During one session, Perls recalled an earlier trauma, and they both realized that Rolfing could release stored physical or emotional trauma. Indeed, some people go through Rolfing to do just that.

If you are in acute pain, Rolfing may not be a good idea because it is a more active and aggressive therapy than some others. It is particularly important to discuss this with your doctor before trying it.

MAGNETIC THERAPY

Although magnetic therapy has been used and debated since medieval times, it has recently become a craze among fitness buffs as a noninvasive way to relieve pain. Static magnets, the kind used on refrigerators or in a magnetic compass, have a magnetic field that does not need replenishing. Advocates of magnetic therapy say magnets have an effect on charged particles in the blood, helping blood vessels to expand and thereby increase circulation. In turn, that increased circulation promotes healing. Some research seems to indicate that magnets do affect ions of compounds carried in the blood. It appears that ions crisscross between the north and south poles of the magnet, causing the blood vessel to widen.

Not all magnets have this effect because they vary in strength and shape. Generally, concentric-circle magnets are recommended and are used just as you would a heating pad.

Place the magnet over the painful area and secure it with tape or an elastic bandage. Then forget about it.

The other type of magnetic therapy is electromagnetic therapy, whereby a machine is used to direct at the patient an alternating electromagnetic field. An example of that would be transcutaneous nerve stimulation or TENS, which is widely used in traditional physical therapy.

✄ NUTRITIONAL THERAPIES

Many books have been written on diets to improve your health. This section is intended to give you an idea of some of the options you have if you decide to explore nutrition and its effects on your health. None of the discussions that follow includes a magic bullet of what to eat to eliminate RSI, but it does include foods that may help ease your symptoms.

First and most importantly, a good diet is the basis for good health. Although experts disagree on exactly what constitutes a good diet, it is fairly well accepted that it is better to consume more whole foods than processed foods and to avoid or limit caffeine and sugar. Beyond that, specifics vary wildly. The best rule of thumb: moderation. Don't eat or drink to excess. If you do on occasion, don't beat yourself up. Having a good diet is not a test, but it can be a building block for your recovery.

Food Philosophies

Food philosophies run the gamut, from protein lovers and carbohydrate lovers to everything in between. No one solution can work for everyone because we each have individual—and changing—relationships with food.

Vegetarians and weight-loss experts are probably familiar with the concept of food combining. The idea is that certain foods, when eaten together, complement each other and maximize their nutritive value. For example, eating rice and beans together is regarded as an efficient combination. The idea has a scientific basis: Different enzymes take a different amount of time to digest various foods.

An Eastern approach to combining foods is based on the principle of yin and yang, a balance of the feminine and masculine. Yin foods are those grown above ground, with high water content; they are soft and juicy. Yang foods tend to be made up of parts of plants grown below ground, like roots and seeds. Macrobiotics is a diet based on the yin-and-yang concept, with an emphasis on whole grains, seeds, and plant foods. The goal is to eat in a way that maintains balance in your body.

Elimination diets are used to find out whether you have food allergies or intolerances. Such a diet should be done only under a doctor's supervision. Typically, it begins with a limited menu, and then gradually, individual foods are introduced to see if you have a reaction to any. Significant food allergies are not that common; but if you have one, it could be compromising your immune system—which needs to operate at optimal efficiency for your general health.

Fasting is used by some who feel a need to cleanse their systems. Some people believe that true healing cannot take place until their system has been cleansed of toxins. Fasting does not mean eliminating all foods and liquids; instead, if you fast, you eliminate solid foods for a specified period of time but continue to drink liquids regularly. There are a variety of fasts, but none should be undertaken for more than a short period of time—for example, no more than two days—without a doctor's supervision.

Targeting RSI

The suggestions that follow are not meant as a prescription for pain or as a substitute for medical treatment. No one food or supplement will make your RSI go away—but some may help ease your symptoms. The suggestions here should be seen as nothing more than a complement to a good, healthy diet and to a good medical treatment program. Again, if you try any of the following, tell your doctor.

Carpal Tunnel Syndrome

As mentioned in a previous chapter, studies have indicated that a deficiency of vitamin B_6 may be linked to carpal tunnel syndrome. Indications are that sufferers may lack sufficient pyridoxine, the largest component of B_6, although no definitive studies show a causal relationship. There is some debate on this point. It is clear that B vitamins are essential to nerve function; what is less clear is how taking them eases carpal tunnel syndrome.

Taking up to 100 milligrams a day of B_6, in combination with a vitamin B complex (which helps increase the absorption of B_6), is most often recommended. It is best to get the specific dosages recommended by a nutritionist. Vitamin B_6 is a water-soluble vitamin, meaning it flushes out of your system so that you don't have to worry about a toxic buildup—as you do with other vitamins. However, if you take too much of it, it may cause nerve damage.

Most of us think of vitamins as benign, and they are, when taken properly. Don't overdo it. You *can* get too much of a good thing.

Another way to try to get more B_6 is simply to eat foods rich in it, like lean meat, fish, poultry, eggs, and dairy products. Because B_6 is likely to be destroyed by high heat, it is not a bad idea to eat as many raw foods as possible, like nuts and seeds (both of which contain a great deal of B_6), and fruits and vegetables.

Another piece of nutritional advice for people with carpal tunnel syndrome is to avoid sodium. Such sodium-rich foods, of course, promote water retention, which can exacerbate your symptoms. If you are pregnant and have symptoms of carpal tunnel syndrome, check any dietary changes with your doctor. Symptoms will often disappear after you have the baby. (Other RSI symptoms may actually improve with pregnancy because of the increased elasticity of muscles and tendons, and hormone production.)

To achieve relief from pain and swelling, try eating half of a fresh pineapple each day for up to three weeks. Fresh pineapple contains bromelain, which has been found to reduce pain and swelling.

Tendinitis and Bursitis

Some experts recommend taking calcium and magnesium supplements together because they are vital for tissue and muscle repair. Magnesium, particularly in magnesium chelate form, is important for connective tissue, while calcium promotes proper muscular function. Once again, dosages should be checked with your nutritionist and/or doctor.

Some nutritionists highly recommend antioxidants, a group of vitamins, minerals, and enzymes that helps protect the body from substances which can impair the immune system, cause infections, and accelerate degenerative diseases. In addition, it is believed that antioxidants help clean out excess lactic-acid buildup in tissues caused by muscle overexertion.

Some common nutrients that act as antioxidants are vita-

min A, which promotes growth and repair of body tissue; vitamin C, which helps maintain the integrity of the immune system; zinc, which functions in wound healing and plays a role in
the body's ability to fight infections; and selenium, which helps
preserve tissue elasticity. Others are beta carotene, vitamin E,
and manganese. The antioxidants appear to work together, so it
is not possible to substitute one for the other. Rather than taking them separately, it's more convenient to take a supplement
or pills that provide a balance of antioxidants.

A variety of natural anti-inflammatory agents can ease
pain and swelling, from black currant oil (which comes in pill
form) to proteolytic enzymes. Or you could try eating half a
fresh pineapple a day, as mentioned.

Avoid or limit alcohol because it causes dehydration,
which can exacerbate pain if you are in an acute phase. In addition, alcohol can interfere with sleep; it reduces stage four
sleep, which is needed for a good rest. Caffeine should be limited as well because it constricts blood vessels, which interferes
with circulation.

Fibromyalgia

Some alternative health specialists believe an imbalance in your
diet can contribute to fibromyalgia. They recommend that you
reduce your intake of refined and processed foods and increase
your consumption of complex carbohydrates. Cut out foods
with artificial additives and sugars. Cutting out sugar, in particular, is easier said than done because it's not always obvious
that some foods contain sugar. Read the labels carefully.

You might also try taking a multivitamin complex that
contains vitamins C and B complex, along with zinc. Some
preliminary research indicates that taking antioxidants may
help as well.

Raynaud's Disease

Because Raynaud's disease is a circulatory disorder, some nutritional experts recommend taking vitamin E: It has been shown to improve circulation. Calcium, magnesium, and zinc may also be recommended.

In addition, avoid fried and fatty foods and caffeine. Stay away from drugs that constrict blood vessels, such as birth control pills.

✖
ONE CAUTION

Remember, there are con artists everywhere. Anyone suffering from a chronic illness or injury would love to have a magic bullet—and there are unscrupulous people ready to take advantage of that. Beware of people who say they can cure you in a few weeks and insist that *only* they possess the means to do it. Stay away from people who try to talk you into spending an exorbitant amount of money. Don't even listen to people who try to tell you that traditional doctors want to keep you sick so they can make more money.

Alternative medicine isn't a bunch of baloney. You may find elements of it that help you. As always, be a careful and informed consumer. Pay attention to your instincts; if something makes you uneasy, there's probably a good reason. But once you get past any cons and shams, exploring alternative medicine can be an informative and fascinating experience.

For computer programmer John, his journey through alternative therapies was an experience that changed his life. "I realized I had to do it myself, from within," he says. He did, with the help of alternative therapies.

CHAPTER 10

COPING WITH
DAY-TO-DAY TASKS

*Several union activists had organized an evening
meeting to discuss workplace safety; the focus was on
RSI. They had invited a range of people, including
several people with severe RSI, and had brought in
pizza and cans of soda for dinner. As people were
passing around the cans, one woman who was wearing splints casually asked the person next to her to
open the can for her. A union steward stared at her
and asked, "You can't do that?"*

*Before she could answer, another woman with
RSI laughed bitterly and said, "Of course, she can't do
that! I can't, either! And I can't open doors or jars!"*

*Stunned, the union steward said quietly, "But I
thought having RSI just meant that you can't type."*

ROUTINE NO LONGER ROUTINE

For most people, RSI does mean having to cut down their typing or simply changing the way they work. But for people seriously debilitated by it, RSI means not being able to do routine chores. It's bad enough to not be able to work but to not be able to take care of yourself at home can be devastating. "That's the piece that hits people real hard," says John Hung, a Minneapolis clinical psychologist who has treated many patients with RSI.

There are ways to do what doctors and occupational therapists call "activities of daily living." It may mean approaching the task differently or getting a simple tool to help you do it. Either way, these approaches can improve the quality of your life dramatically while you are working on getting better. "It's amazing how many things require the use of your hands," says one man, who has had RSI on and off for seven years.

Remember to keep your expectations realistic. And try not to be too upset by the unpredictable ways in which RSI can interfere with your life, whether it's not being able to turn on a washing machine or being unable to open a locker door. Those experiences can be upsetting, but they can also be a spur to finding creative solutions. Following are some practical suggestions for coping with the tasks most people do every day without even thinking about them.

HOUSEHOLD CHORES

Housework

If you can afford it, hire help. If keeping a clean house is important to you, it's well worth it. If you can't afford it, consider bartering for it. One woman traded computer training (ironi-cally) for housework. Some insurance plans will pay for household help. It can't hurt to ask.

Asking family members to pick up the slack can be hard. They may be feeling resentful of your injury, burdened them-selves, and scared. Even though you are the one who is in-jured, they have feelings about your RSI they may not even be able to express. Those feelings can easily come out in argu-ments over housework. If you find yourself in such a situation, spare yourself the fireworks, and get help elsewhere.

Conversely, some family members may take over house-work completely. One woman, a bookkeeper so debilitated by RSI that she was unable to work, admitted she was rather en-joying her injury because her husband and children were fi-nally doing a lot more of the chores around the house. That may be fine for a while, but, ultimately, it's not fair to you or your family. You have little incentive to get better if you are en-joying being taken care of. It's far better to negotiate a com-promise in which everyone's needs are met.

If you feel up to doing housework, you can build up the grips on mops and brooms by wrapping them with weather stripping, for example. That enables you to use them without having to grip them so tightly. You can do the same thing to faucets, which can be painful to turn. Reachers and special brushes are available in specialty catalogs. (A list of catalogs featuring adaptive aids is in the appendix.)

Try to pace yourself. Marion, who has returned to work after two carpal tunnel surgeries, manages her housework now by not doing it all in one day. She says she's had to learn to live with more mess, but that it's worth it because she avoids a lot of pain later. "I've come to the point where I just accept the house the way it is," she says.

Cooking

Get takeout food. Buy prepared foods at the grocery store. Buy garlic that is already chopped, and cheese that is already shredded. Go out to eat. It costs a little more, but it's worth it. To save your hands from doing dishes, consider paper plates. Use Silverstone or Teflon-coated pans to reduce the amount of scrubbing. Let dishes air-dry.

For people who love to cook, the inability to use their hands to cook can be a particular emotional blow. Remember: This is only temporary.

If you can do some cooking, use smaller containers to hold your food to minimize the amount of weight you must lift. If you need to move a pot or container from one part of the kitchen to another, use a potholder to slide it across. Use small containers to freeze food. It's much easier to get ice cubes out of an ice tray if you only fill the tray half full.

As anyone with RSI who tries to cook knows, chopping food can be painful if not impossible. There is, however, a wide array of special tools available to help you cook. For example, some knives are designed for ease of use and maneuverability. One type has a handle like a pistol grip, specifically designed to take the pressure off your arm while cutting. Another knife is weighted so that even if your strength is limited, you can use it easily. In addition, there are entire lines of cooking utensils with oversize handles designed for easier gripping. There are also well-designed peelers that enable you to peel potatoes or apples without putting too much strain on your hands. All these tools can take much of the pain out of chopping, slicing, and dicing.

There are holders for milk cartons that make it much easier to pull a carton out of the refrigerator. There are openers for jars and bottles, ranging from a rubber disc to a Y-shaped opener. And there are spring-loaded loop scissors that almost eliminate the pressure needed to cut something. For drinking soda, there are soda can tab grabbers. All are available in specialty catalogs (see the appendix). In addition, if you are seeing an occupational therapist, he may have demos to try.

There are makeshift adaptations you can use around your kitchen. Put items you use most frequently on a lazy Susan. Strap a belt loop on the refrigerator door handle to make it easier to open. Do the same with cabinet drawers that are difficult to open. If you have room, open shelving for storage is much easier on the hands. Store heavy things you need to use where you can easily slide rather than lift them.

Many small appliances can make your life easier, such as an electric can opener, food processor, battery-operated flour sifter, or toaster oven. One woman with RSI who loved to bake splurged and bought herself a bread maker. She and her family loved the aroma of bread baking.

❋
PERSONAL CARE

Being unable to take care of your personal needs can be humiliating. Again, there are ways to cope.

Build up the faucets in the bathroom with weather stripping or rubber tubing to make them easier to turn. Build up your toothbrush the same way. Get toothpaste in a pump dispenser. Special nail clippers are available in specialty catalogs. Use a lightweight hair dryer. Put an ergonomically designed door handle on your bathroom door to make the knob easier to turn. Don't buy shampoos or conditioners in containers that you have to squeeze.

In getting dressed, choose clothes with the least amount of fuss—that is, fewer buttons and zippers. If you have trouble fastening buttons, there are button fasteners available in specialty catalogs. Pulling on pantyhose can be excruciating; opt for pants when possible. Skirts with elastic waists and undergarments with Velcro fasteners can make life easier.

Some people with RSI dread winter not only because the cold is hard on their symptoms but because they have to put on heavy coats and jackets. If possible, dress in layers. If wearing gloves is impossible because you wear splints, wear mittens. And, think summer.

Don't let yourself go. It's important to take care of your appearance. It feels good to look good. One woman who had had long hair all her life found it just too hard to deal with after she got RSI. Reluctantly, she decided to cut it short. To her surprise, she found she looked better.

✖

GETTING AROUND

Opening Doors

Opening a door is something few able-bodied people think about; but if you have painful RSI, it can consume much thought and energy. Try pushing doors open with your hip or shoulder (*if* you don't have a problem with your shoulder). Remember, however, that using muscles for tasks they're not designed to do can cause aches and pains in different parts of your body. If you do this, try alternating the hip or shoulder you use.

Two friends with RSI had a buddy system whenever they went out. If they were about to leave a restaurant, they waited until they saw someone else headed for the door so they could slip in behind that person. If they couldn't do that, they took turns bumping open doors for each other.

For doors at home, put special handles over doorknobs to make it easier to open them. Just as useful is a key holder that slips over your keys. That can eliminate the pain that comes from the seemingly simple action of twisting a key to open your door.

Driving

Opening a car window manually or twisting a steering wheel can be particularly painful for someone with acute RSI. For driving a car, automate as much as possible. That means getting a car that has power steering, power windows, and power-seat controls. Consider getting a car-door opener as well. If you drive a stick shift, you may have to give it up.

If you already own a car and are not in a financial position to buy a new one, try building up your steering wheel with a material like lambs wool so that you don't have to grip it so tightly. If holding the wheel is still difficult, you can get what's called a *spinner knob* (also known as a *necker's knob* because it permitted a boy to put his arm around his date while driving). A spinner knob is not legal in every state so you may have to obtain a special restriction on your driver's license to use one, but it can make it easier for you to drive.

Again, a key holder for car keys makes it easier to turn the ignition. A variety is available in catalogs. If you have trouble turning your neck, consider putting a wide-angled mirror in the car.

You may be able to get some of the equipment you need for free. Your insurance company may pay for it, or you could contact local vocational rehabilitation agencies. Many such agencies have counselors who help adapt cars and vans for the disabled.

When driving, don't grip the wheel tightly. And forget what you were taught in driving class: Don't hold the wheel in the classic "10 and 2 position" (or even in the new "3 and 9" position that is recommended if you have an airbag). It's easier on your hands and arms to hold the steering wheel at the base.

Finally, when you want to park the car in the garage (if you have one), get a garage-door opener. They are inexpensive and relatively easy to install.

Traveling

One man with RSI confessed that he had canceled a long-planned trip because he knew that he wouldn't be able to haul his luggage through airports. And he knew other people would think he was "weird" if he asked for help.

Traveling with RSI can be tough. Getting around with luggage can seem like an insurmountable task. So can merely riding in a car, train, or bus. For some, the vibration and being forced to sit in a constrained position can set off symptoms. For others, who are already worn down by RSI, making the connections needed on a long trip can simply be too exhausting.

One way to cope with luggage is to get a carrier on wheels so that you can drag it as much as possible. Most airports have skycaps who will handle your luggage for you. The same is true for some hotels. The fact is, if you need help like that, you won't be able to travel as cheaply as you might like. It's a trade-off.

When flying, try to get a seat with as much legroom as possible. Walk around during the flight. Try to avoid making a flight with a lot of connections. Make the travel as easy on yourself as possible.

❧
WORKING AT HOME

Even if you are out of work, use tools at home to take care of tasks like paying bills or setting up appointments. Electrify where you can. Get an electric stapler, letter opener, or stamping machine. Here are some other tips.

Telephone

Holding a telephone receiver for more than a few minutes can be exhausting for someone with severe RSI. A headset is cheap and easy to use (and will enable you to stay on the phone much longer!). Or try a speakerphone. Some people don't like them because of the hollow sound, but they are a way to ease the wear and tear on your neck and arms.

Use the redial button for frequently called numbers. If you have an answering machine with the capacity to save messages, use that function to avoid writing notes, if writing is painful.

If pushing buttons is painful, try using a pen or pencil instead of your fingers. There are also phones with larger keypads that require less pressure to push the buttons.

Writing

Writing can be one of the most frustrating and painful tasks because you need to do it so often. Try building up your pen with pen grips or moleskin. Or get an ergonomically designed fat pen, which is widely available and can ease the strain writing puts on your hands.

If you need to do more than write notes at home, put a pad on every desk or other surface you use so that your hands and arms don't press against a sharp edge. And if you need to work at home, set up your workstation following the guidelines outlined in chapter 5.

Reading

Reading for work or pleasure can be hard because it can cause you pain to bend your neck if you are, for example, trying to read in bed. Or, you may find a book too heavy to lift or the fine-motor movement of turning pages too painful. There are book stands that make it simple to slide the book into a convenient spot to read it. There are also page turners that strap on your arms; they stick to the pages, enabling you to turn them more easily.

Switching on lamps can send shooting pains up the arms for any sufferer, and lamp-switch extensions levers are available to minimize that pain.

Opening the Mail

Opening the mail is such a mundane task, but it can be excruciatingly painful to someone with RSI. Use spring-loaded loop scissors, which are easier on the hands than trying to rip open the mail with your thumb and fingers.

SHOPPING

First and foremost, forget bulk-buying. When shopping for necessities like food, buy in smaller amounts that are easier to carry. It costs a little more, but it saves significant wear and tear on your arms. In addition, shop more often so that you have less to carry. Some people with RSI have their groceries delivered.

If you must buy medications, ask your pharmacist to give them to you with caps that are *not* childproof so that you can avoid painful twisting. If you forget to ask the pharmacist, there are pill-cap openers you can get to open the bottle without hurting yourself.

Carrying anything can cause pain. In some grocery stores, clerks are available to help carry packages. Or, if your shoulders do not bother you, try wearing a backpack to carry items. Even if you don't have shoulder problems, avoid using a shoulder bag. Excessive weight on one shoulder can contribute to thoracic outlet syndrome. Put essentials in a fanny pack. Other things, like an umbrella, can be held by a belt loop.

Betsy, a free-lance writer who was fifty-four when she was injured, recalls somewhat ruefully that her parents had to help her shop for groceries when she was unable to do it herself. She felt deeply uncomfortable about it, sure that other people in the store were thinking, "What is that woman doing letting her aged parents carry everything around?"

But she had no choice; she needed help.

SLEEPING

Even sleeping can be a problem if you have RSI. Try arranging pillows to support your neck and arms in a neutral, comfortable position. This may take some experimenting and a couple of extra pillows, but you'll likely find a position that works. You probably don't need to buy an expensive orthopedic pillow to do this.

CHILD CARE

If you have an infant, you will, of course, want to hold the baby as much as possible. Not all baby carriers are easy on your shoulders, however. Some are designed to take the weight off your shoulders and spread it across your body, making it much easier to handle the weight. They are specifically advertised as beijng designed for taking the weight off your shoulders and back, and are available through many baby product catalogs

Whenever possible, use pillows to support your hands and arms. If you are breast-feeding, get a nursing pillow. They're cheap, easy to use, and take enormous strain off your arms, neck, and shoulders. They're also available in baby-product catalogs. If you need to pump breast milk, consider renting an electric pump. They are relatively inexpensive if you rent them for several months and are far easier on your hands than manual or battery-operated pumps.

Diaper bags can be just as bad as a shoulder bag. There is a diaper bag that you can strap around your waist like a fanny pack and it holds just about as much as a standard diaper bag. It also provides a convenient ledge on which to rest your baby.

If you have the room, a changing table is worth the investment in order to eliminate unnecessary bending or reaching. As your child grows older, you may have to switch to the floor, however. One woman who found that she couldn't lift her daughter as she got bigger set up changing stations on the floor in her baby's room and throughout the house so that she could avoid painful lifting.

If you suffer from RSI, picking up a baby by hooking your thumbs under their armpits can be excruciatingly painful. Try putting one hand under the baby's bottom instead.

If you have older children, try to explain to them why you can't do certain things. Encourage them to do things on their own.

❀
PERSONAL SAFETY

RSI can elicit fears about personal safety that you might not have thought about before. You may feel especially vulnerable if you wear splints and it is obvious to others that you are disabled. Avoiding problems is a matter of using common sense.

When you are walking somewhere, especially at night, stay away from buildings and doorways and try to stick to well-lit areas. Have your key ready when you approach your car or front door. When possible, travel with a companion.

If you do a lot of driving, consider getting a cellular phone. Set it up with an autodialer, and use a telephone holder for it. A cellular phone can be invaluable if your car breaks down. At stop signs and traffic lights, keep the car in gear. Keep any packages or bags in your trunk. And always keep your car doors locked.

❀
HOBBIES

You may have a hobby that exacerbates your injury. Some cited by people with RSI include woodworking, gardening, playing the piano, and sewing. If it is something important to you, you may be able to continue doing it, but consider doing less of it, or getting help. For example, you might be able to get a friend to till your garden, but then you could still plant seeds and water it.

If your hobby causes significant pain, consider giving it up, even if it's only temporarily. One man had to give up playing the piano and doing crossword puzzles. A woman had to stop painting. It can be hard to let go of something that gives you pleasure, but you may find other things that you enjoy as much.

SOCIALIZING

A crowded setting can be uncomfortable if you are in acute pain. One man remembers being exhausted after going to see a highly touted art exhibit at a major museum. He tensed his muscles as people crowded next to him to look at the art. By the end of the exhibit, he said, "I was ready to go to bed!"

Parties can be a problem if people try to greet you with a slap on the back or a big, friendly bear hug. John, the former computer programmer from San Francisco, used to head off people from shaking hands with him by wearing splints when he went out. "It worked," he says.

Eating a meal with a friend or a date can be embarrassing if you have trouble cutting food. Try to order food that doesn't need cutting, like pasta, pizza, or salad. But if you find yourself in a jam, don't be afraid to ask your companion or the waiter for a little help. Most people are eager to help.

Entertaining is probably too big a job to take on alone because of the work involved. It really requires a lot of physical labor. If you want to throw a party, get help. Potluck parties are easy, and most people enjoy pitching in.

✤
GIFTS

One woman who found it painful to do nearly anything with her hands used to dread receiving care packages from her sister, who lived in another city. Her sister always thoughtfully packed up articles on RSI and any other items she thought would be helpful and sent them off in a box with all the edges tightly taped. "Just opening those boxes was a nightmare," the woman says. "I would groan every time I got one."

Another woman who regularly wore splints because of severe tendinitis and carpal tunnel syndrome recalls the shock she felt the day she opened a birthday gift sent by a relative in another city. It was a heavy silver bracelet. It was a gift she couldn't even consider putting on, even if she didn't wear splints, because the bracelet's weight would have been too much for her inflamed arms. Although almost everyone has received an inappropriate or thoughtless gift, she couldn't believe that her complaints about her arms had apparently failed to register with her family. She couldn't muster any enthusiasm to thank her relative for the gift, which left the relative angry and confused.

In short, gifts, even from the most well-intentioned relatives and friends, can cause unexpected problems. What's the best way to handle receiving them? It's up to you, but you're probably better off saying nothing.

In giving gifts, don't wrap them in elaborate wrapping or bows. Use gift-wrap services in your department stores, or place them in an unusual container. Remember, it's the thought—not the wrapping—that counts. Of course, the easiest thing to do is to shop by catalog; mail-order companies will wrap and send the gift.

✂
GETTING BACK TO WORK

If you have been forced to take time off from work because of RSI, returning to your job means an adjustment, even if you've been out only a short time. You not only have to change the way you work but you have to deal with the attitudes of coworkers. Before doing anything, however, you must determine when you're physically ready to return.

When Are You Ready?

Your doctor should determine when you are ready to return to work. He is likely to base such a decision on a physical examination and reading of therapists' reports. In some cases, a doctor may order a functional-capacity exam, which is designed to determine your muscle strength and capacity, and to identify your specific limits.

Before you return to work, you will need a doctor's note. It should specify how much time you can work and what tasks you can and cannot do. Specifying "light duty" is not enough. Your doctor needs to understand the physical tasks your job entails in order to set appropriate limits. That is not only for your benefit, but for your employer's as well.

Your own attitude—and that of your employer—will also be important in judging your readiness to return to work. If you are eager and have a sympathetic employer willing to make accommodations, your doctor is likely to be more positive. If your employer is unsympathetic, your doctor may be hesitant. Sometimes a patient who is fearful about returning to work needs a nudge from a doctor; other times, an overly eager patient needs to be held back. There are no hard-and-fast rules on the right time to return to work.

Go Back Slowly

When you and your doctor decide the time is right for you, *go back slowly.*

You may think you feel much better, but part of that perception is due to the fact that you haven't been doing what hurt you in the first place. Don't try to do too much too soon. Even if it feels silly, pace yourself. That means limiting the hours you spend at the job, as well as the hours you spend on a keyboard. If you can, do other tasks that aren't as taxing on your hands and arms. Some companies familiar with RSI have come up with temporary alternative work for employees with RSI.

A sympathetic employer will understand. The doctor should outline a patient's physical capacities, and the employee and employer need to enable the patient to work within those capacities. If you have an unsympathetic employer, point to your doctor's note, which delineates your limits—and stick to them. If you have a union, talk to your representative to help gain the accommodations you need. (More on your legal rights will be discussed in chapter 13.)

Gradually, you'll find yourself getting stronger and able to do more things. Rehabilitation specialists call this *work hardening.* The length of time it takes varies. It can take from a few weeks to as long as three months in severe cases. Expect setbacks. Anytime you try something new, you are working new muscles and can expect some pain and soreness. Some soreness is tolerable; burning pain is not.

Dealing with Coworkers

Dealing with skeptical coworkers can be tough. There are often established channels through which you can approach a supervisor, but they are less established with coworkers. (Employer reactions to RSI, of course, vary. Ways to deal with your employer will be discussed in greater depth in a later chapter.) Every workplace has internal politics. Your coworkers may decide that it's not politic to be associating with someone who has filed for worker's compensation, for example. That's hard to fight. "You find out who your real friends are," says Melita, a Minneapolis-based production manager who has been out of work since 1991 because of her injury.

People with RSI often talk about the sense of betrayal they feel if and when their coworkers or supervisor don't believe them. Career is so much a part of our lives, of our personal identities, that to lose the ability to work and then to be seen as a malingerer can be a crushing blow. Again, talk to people who understand and carry on with your recovery and your life. There won't be much you can do about people who persist in thinking that your RSI is not real. "It's too close to home," Melita says. "People don't want to believe it because it could easily happen to them."

Changing the Way You Work

Changing the way you work may be as simple as getting a different piece of equipment, or as fundamental as changing your attitude. Getting the equipment is likely to be a lot easier than changing your attitude. If you are a hard worker, as many people with RSI are, it's difficult to do less or slow down. Your own self-image may be tied to your ability to work hard. If you are careful, you will be able to accomplish as much without hurting yourself. You don't have to do everything you did before.

Sometimes it's a matter of setting limits with your boss. Even if you have a sympathetic employer, he may not understand that asking you to stay late or do "a little extra typing" will hurt you. It's not easy, but you need to assert yourself and explain your limits. Or, volunteer to do another task that won't hurt you. Sometimes your boss will understand, other times he won't.

Working is an adjustment because when you are home and feel your symptoms flare up, you can stop what you're doing, rest, and ice the painful area. At work, this isn't so easy. But most offices and plants have refrigerators where you can store ice packs or a cup filled with frozen water. If you feel your symptoms flare up while you're on the job, take a break and ice. Don't work through pain.

You'll need to make some changes in equipment when you return to work. Most of what you'll need is inexpensive and should be paid for by your employer. (In setting up a computer workstation, follow the guidelines suggested in chapter 5.) In addition, consider getting some of the tools mentioned earlier, such as an electric stapler, letter opener, or stamping machine. To deal with heavy files in file cabinets, try weaving plastic ties through the tops of hanging files to create a handle that's easier to grip.

For some people, typing is too painful to do even after returning to work. A voice-activated computer is one option. They have become more sophisticated—and much less expensive—in recent years. Many users swear by them.

Al, a staff writer at the *Minneapolis Star and Tribune*, turned to a voice-activated computer after finding that typing his regular column was too painful. His doctor initially prescribed thumb splints to minimize the intense pain at the base of his thumbs. "The joke among my friends was that I should use the space bar less and use big words," he says.

He gets along well using his Dragon Dictate, but he says one downside is that chewing sounds confuse the computer so he can no longer eat while typing. He laughs at the occasional *wordo*, his term for the inevitable wrong words that result from using this kind of technology. Here are some samples of some of the computer's early unedited goofs of familiar passages before it got to know his voice:

The Raven

"Once upon a midnight jury, well I powder, week
*   and very,*

Over many a right and serious volume of
*   forthcoming more"*

Lincoln's Gettysburg Address

"For store and seven years ago our fathers wrote
fourth on this content a new nation, embassy in
liberty and education to the protozoan that all
them are created people."

The Star-Spangled Banner

"Old say can you see by the tongs early late,

What so probably we pale at the college last cleaning,

Whose broad strikes and great store, through the
*   parallels five*

Or the reference we watch were so talented string?"

Al says that for another column, he might read aloud "some complete garbage" like the *Congressional Record* or the fine print on his credit-card bill and "see whether the computer turns it into Shakespeare."

Joking aside, Al finds that he must think more about a sentence before writing it, but generally, says the voice-activated technology is easy to use. And, even after several years of using it, he is still "amazed by the technology."

CHAPTER 11

RIDING THE EMOTIONAL ROLLER COASTER

Linda, a dental hygienist, had worked for thirty years when it happened. She began dropping things and accidentally cut patients while cleaning their teeth. The pain and weakness got so bad that her doctor told her to stop everything— "no straightening up, no cooking, no opening doors," Linda says. That left the burden of household chores to her teenage son because as a single mother without disability insurance, she couldn't afford help. "We're poor. We're hanging onto our apartment by a thread."

A lawyer persuaded Linda that her injury was work-related and that she should file for worker's compensation, which she did, "out of desperation." To her astonishment, her employer, whom she regarded as a friend, fought her claim. "I still can't believe that he doesn't believe me," she says.

Linda has had to give up work, hobbies, and anything but the bare essentials. One day, she and her son argued over housework. Something "snapped," Linda says, and she took an overdose of pills. Her son called 911 and she was rushed to the hospital. Linda is trying to get back on track, but still struggles with the pain and physical limitations caused by her RSI.

EMOTIONAL ISSUES

Linda was dealing with other personal issues along with RSI, and, clearly, they all came to a head the day she tried to commit suicide. But her story paints a stark picture of the emotional devastation that can be caused, at least in part, by a chronic injury such as RSI. Though most sufferers don't face such extreme circumstances, many do experience the same emotions. RSI thrusts people onto a roller coaster of emotions that friends, family, and people treating them often don't understand. But patients who've had it for a while, and therapists who've treated them, say there are some phases many people experience—denial, panic and fear, guilt and/or shame, anger, grieving and/or depression, and acceptance.

Each phase needs to be understood as normal and an important step toward healing. There is no set beginning or end to each phase; in fact, you may find yourself "cycling" in and out of them for a while. But as your recovery progresses, you will work your way through the emotional issues. Paying attention to them is as important as paying attention to your physical recovery because the two go hand in hand.

RSI is different from other chronic injuries because of the ongoing discovery of loss, says John Hung, Ph.D., a Minneapolis clinical psychologist who has treated many patients with RSI. Because RSI makes simple tasks impossible, you are constantly reminded of your physical limitations. Peeling a potato or lifting a book are examples of minor physical tasks that we take for granted. Discovering that you can no longer do such things is a shock.

Remember, too, that your hands and arms are a means of expression, creativity, nurturance, and love. To lose the use of your hands and arms is a severe blow to your sense of self. It is difficult for people who have not experienced such a loss to understand its profound emotional impact.

Each of us copes with trauma and loss differently. Because it is so difficult, consider talking to others with RSI (to be discussed in more detail later in this chapter). Friends and loved ones may not have the understanding and/or skills to help you with the confusing emotions. A support system of people that truly understands what it's like can help immensely. You may not experience every phase described here, or in the precise order described, but don't be surprised if you do. RSI is a profound trauma.

❋
PHASES OF RSI

Denial

Denial is a common first reaction to bad news and is, in fact, a normal and healthy defense mechanism. It makes it easier to handle an emergency or to cope with a crisis. Unfortunately, with RSI, denial can be dangerous. The longer you deny that you have a problem, the greater your risk of more serious physical injury.

This is a difficult phase because most people aren't conscious of the fact that they're doing it (hence the term *denial*).

The injury itself is hard to pin down: The pains may come and go, and doctors don't always recognize RSI. And if your doctor isn't worried, why should you be?

Theo, an Australian journalist who has reported stories all over the world, recalls hearing complaints from secretaries about RSI; they brushed it off. "We would go to a pub after work, and we would say this was only for women," he says. Then, in 1987, while throwing a ball for his dog, "I got this extraordinary pain down my arm. Thinking it was a muscle pull, I went on." The pain continued, but Theo says he "was stoic. I was macho." A year later, he couldn't brush his teeth. Though he has since gotten his injury under control, he regrets his long months of stoicism.

"There are few people who face it in its early stages," says Susan Nobel, a social worker who runs a support group for people with RSI at the Mt. Sinai-Irving J. Selikoff Occupational and Environmental Medicine Center in New York. "Those who do, do better."

Psychologist Hung agrees, but points out that facing up to the injury is a difficult adjustment for most people. "Even after they've reconciled themselves to the fact that this is here to stay, there's the issue of the magnitude of it," he says.

To be confronted by your physical limitations on a daily basis is not easy. Denial is one way to cope. It can take several forms, Hung says. Some people minimize the injury, calling it a strain. Others minimize the physical limitations it has caused, insisting on continuing activities that may exacerbate RSI. Still others downplay the emotional impact of the loss.

Studies have shown RSI afflicts the hardest workers; for them, it is particularly hard to slow down or give up their work. And there is little social support for people who can't work as hard as they used to—or can't work at all. We live in a society that does not easily tolerate disability.

Most people initially deny or minimize RSI because it can be a terrifying injury. It brings you face-to-face with your own physical limitations and, in a sense, your own mortality. That very real blow to your self-esteem, to your sense of self, would be overwhelming without the emotional defense of denial.

Add to all this the practical and very real fear of losing your job. Many employers still do not understand RSI or believe that it's real; stories of people losing their jobs because of RSI abound. This is a difficult issue. It's not easy to find another job, particularly if you are limited by such an injury. But the fact is, you can't replace your hands and arms. You won't win any brownie points if you work until you can't physically move.

RSI is not caused by a sudden or dramatic accident, like being hit by a car or falling down a flight of stairs. Either of these tragedies would certainly be more socially acceptable and easier to understand. Instead, most of the time it sneaks up on you. It's hard to believe. It doesn't seem to make sense. "It's very hard to accept that your body is letting you down in this way," social worker Nobel says.

Given these characteristics, it's understandable that people deny and minimize their injury. But the best thing you can do for yourself—and your hands and arms—is to face it. The sooner, the better.

One secretary who developed debilitating RSI kicks herself for not acting sooner. "I should have known better," she says. "So, in that sense, I adopted a head-in-the-sand attitude about it until I physically couldn't move." In fact, she *shouldn't have* known better. RSI is an injury that confounds many people. There is no reason to blame yourself if it has confounded you.

Panic and Fear

Once denial subsides, some people panic. RSI is, after all, a frightening injury with potentially far-reaching consequences for your work and life. If you've seen other people forced out of work by their RSI, it becomes all the more frightening.

One man called a doctor whom he knew his coworkers had seen and insisted on getting an appointment that day. The doctor's secretary, hearing the fear in his voice, tried to schedule him as soon as possible but was only able to offer him an appointment the next day. That wasn't good enough, the man insisted, he needed to see the doctor *today*. Otherwise, he told her, he could lose the use of his arms.

Fortunately, another patient canceled, and she was able to get him in that day. It turned out that his injury was mild. A few small changes to his workstation and some advice about posture took care of his symptoms.

Panic is not always such a bad thing. It can motivate you to act quickly, to seek out the help you need. But it can also exacerbate your symptoms. People tend to tense their muscles when they panic—the classic flight or fight response. The more you tense your muscles, the more pain you'll feel. And the more pain you feel, the more panicked you'll be. It can quickly become a vicious cycle.

This is when it's important to have a doctor who is knowledgeable and reassuring. Although no physician will be able to give you precise answers about how long it will take you to get better, he can give you a sense of the seriousness of your injury and what you need to do to heal.

There is no need to panic. RSI is treatable.

That's not to say that your fears aren't legitimate. They may be. You may face the possible loss of your job or of some income. As one man said, "It rattled me because my financial security and my family's financial security depended on me being able to do my job."

That's significant, but worrying about it will do you little good. You're better off focusing on your recovery. Once you do, other things should begin to fall into place.

Guilt/Shame

Once past the early stages of RSI, it's not uncommon for people to feel guilty—about their limitations, their dependence on others, and being injured in the first place. They worry about coworkers having to take on more work because of them, and they worry that nobody will believe them. Or they may feel shame, worrying about what others think of them. With guilt, people feel they've done something bad.

Tim was injured in his job as a university librarian in Philadelphia. Like many people with RSI, he was juggling many responsibilities at once—his library job, work as a teaching assistant, and graduate studies. When the pain hit him suddenly over the course of a week in 1995, he was "in a bad way." He couldn't hold a cup of tea or twist a doorknob. A doctor diagnosed him with tenosynovitis and cubital tunnel syndrome and advised him to go on light duty. Tim did, but felt guilty, he says. "Everybody is being productive around you, and you're just out of step. You feel like you're shirking your duties." Tim's condition has improved since then, but the memory of that time remains vivid. He recalls feeling like a "traitor, hypochondriac, complainer."

That kind of guilt and shame, according to some therapists, can be a motivator. Such feelings can spur you to find ways to get around your limitations. Someone worried that coworkers suspect he is malingering might find another way to do a job.

However, that isn't always appropriate with RSI. First of all, the injury isn't your fault. You are likely feeling guilty not because you caused your injury but because you are used to being productive, and you want to work. Second, working through pain because you feel guilty about it will only make matters worse.

Carol, a bakery worker in Iowa, worried about shooting pains in her arms but was afraid her bosses were thinking, "What's she trying to pull? Is she trying to get off work or trying to get paid off?" Several of her coworkers shared this worry and avoided reporting their symptoms at all, which only led to more serious problems for them later.

Feeling guilty is understandable, especially if you see your loved ones take on a greater burden because of your limitations. It may not be merely a matter of household chores and child rearing; it may be a financial burden as well. That's hard to take for people who are used to supporting themselves and contributing their share.

Bear in mind, however, that this is only temporary. You will need a little extra help and support for a while. You must be able to ask for help—and that, say many people with RSI, is the hardest thing they had to learn. Dental hygienist Linda has always been someone who helped others. "I love helping others," she says. "I'm not comfortable with being helpless and it being reversed."

With RSI, you have no choice. Asking for help takes practice, Nobel says. "I think that if people ask for help in a nonwhining way, they will get help because people like to help people."

There is no reason to feel guilty about accepting a little help from others. In fact, one unconscious reason for feeling guilty and ashamed of RSI is that, deep down, some people may want to be taken care of for a while. This is especially true for people who are used to shouldering much of the responsibility in their work or personal lives—exactly the kind of people who often get RSI. Such people have disavowed their own feelings of dependency and worry that if others find out they have such feelings, they'll be ridiculed. That doesn't usually happen; feelings of dependency are normal, especially with RSI. Acknowledging your need for help and the fact that you can't do everything will enable you to move on.

Anger

RSI is fundamentally unfair. A job should not hurt you, and society should not blame you. Unfortunately, both things happen. People suffering from RSI often rage against their employers and their colleagues, who frequently don't, or won't, understand. They talk about the sense of betrayal they feel. They've worked hard, tried to do their best, and suddenly, people don't believe them or, worse, don't care. As Angela, who had worked for twenty years as a secretary when she was afflicted with carpal tunnel syndrome says, "Nobody said, 'I'm sorry.'"

That, says Stephanie Barnes, who runs the Association for Repetitive Motion Syndrome, in California, comes as a blow to many RSI patients. "One of the most painful things is that most people think their boss and coworkers will rally around them," she says. "I think it's one of the biggest shocks when that doesn't happen."

Even for those who have a supportive employer and coworkers, the trials of dealing with worker's compensation, physical therapy, and disability can be infuriating. Getting approval for necessary treatment and benefits can take years.

Social worker Nobel believes anger can be a positive emotion, spurring people to take charge of their health. "It's critical to take charge," she says. She encourages people to be politically active on the issues of RSI and ergonomic regulations as a way to channel their anger.

You may find such activism a good fit for you, or you may not. There are other ways you can use your anger. It may be a matter of asserting yourself with someone who has been rude or insensitive. Small victories can make a difference.

At the same time, unchanneled anger can interfere with your recovery. People tense their muscles when they're angry, causing more spasm, pain, and misery. Hanging onto your anger can cause you to hang onto your pain. Although your anger is certainly justified, it may not be helping you. When it stops helping you, you need to let it go.

That's easier said than done. You may need to let it run its course. It's likely that anyone who tells you that you shouldn't be angry will wind up infuriating you even more. Often, people who are angry over a loss seem demanding and selfish. They may even seem irrational. It is difficult for others to understand the kind of hurt and rage you may be experiencing. The angrier you are, the less likely they are to want to understand. If you find that you are alienating others, you may need to step back and re-evaluate your behavior.

Constantly feeling angry at the world and the unfairness of your injury reflects a fundamental, underlying assumption: Life should be fair. In fact, life is often unfair. If you can accept that fact, your anger is likely to subside, and you'll have more emotional room to accept whatever good things may come your way as a result of your RSI.

You may never be able to let go of your anger completely. Rosa, an engraver who had to give up a job she loved because of RSI, says she is happy now and has been able to go on with her life, "but every once in a while, someone says something, and I feel that little core of anger inside. It never goes away."

Grief/Depression

RSI involves a great deal of loss. It is profound loss, on many levels—a loss of control, the ability to do things you once loved, and the sense of fulfillment that comes from doing a job well. There are more concrete losses as well—the possible loss of a job, income, even friends. Not to mention the loss of the use of your hands, which are central to everything we do. It is natural and healthy to mourn loss, and grieving is a way to do that.

A feeling of sadness or emptiness is a normal response to loss. People with severe RSI often go through a period, or periods, of grief. They are coping with a major trauma and dramatic change in their lives. If they are unable to work because of their injury, they must deal with isolation, a loss of structure, pain, and an inability to function. In addition, they must work at getting better—going to therapy, doing tedious exercises, and remembering to ice or use heat packs when they have a flare-up. None of this is fun. It would be abnormal *not* to grieve.

Yet, friends and even some professionals treating RSI often expect you to keep a positive attitude. It is true that a good, hopeful attitude helps recovery, but it's hard to keep that up consistently in the face of the inevitable setbacks that occur during the process of recovery. Most people don't really want to hear how you feel, nor do they want to hear complaints. Even close friends won't want to hear your complaints over a long period of time. It's not personal; it's just human nature.

You may find yourself feeling very alone. Even well-meaning friends can make hurtful comments. One RSI patient bristled with anger when a friend told her she must be enjoying her "vacation." She later realized that her friend wasn't trying to insult her; it was just that her friend had never been out of work and simply didn't understand.

Sometimes, clinical depression can develop from what has begun as normal grieving. If you have a history of depressive illness in your family, you may be at risk. Signals that your grief has turned to depression include being unable to fall asleep or stay asleep, loss of appetite, feeling pervasively self-critical, and having problems concentrating. You may find yourself stuck in a gloomy, pessimistic mood.

If you experience any or all of those symptoms for more than a few weeks, consult a doctor or mental-health professional with expertise in depression. Clinical depression is an illness that can be as incapacitating as RSI and, worse, life-threatening. It is vital that it be treated.

There may also be a physical component contributing to depression. The same chemicals in the body that serve to mediate pain also mediate depression. People in pain become depressed, and people who are depressed feel more pain. Given all that, brief periods of depression are part of the healing process. Typically, they clear up within a reasonable amount of time. It is when the depression lasts longer than a brief period that you should be concerned.

You may reject the notion that you have a depressive illness by saying to yourself, "But I have a good reason to be depressed." In fact, you do have good reason to feel depressed. There is nothing wrong or bad about feeling sadness and grief over a trauma such as RSI, but don't suffer from a depressive illness needlessly. Clinical depression can be treated. Normal sadness and grief usually respond to the caring of family and friends and the passage of time. Clinical depression does not, and it may well prevent you from reaching the final stage of recovery—acceptance.

Acceptance

Acceptance is the most vital stage for well-being because it paves the way for healing. It is a matter of learning to live with your limitations and welcome some of the changes RSI has brought to your life. Some changes can be positive. One woman speaks with fondness of the new friendships she has made; a man talks with pride about taking better care of his body and soul.

This is the heroic phase. Few people understand what it's like to live with a disability unless they've done it themselves.

Yet people with RSI who have reached the point of accepting their injury show real creativity and courage in dealing with their limitations. It's not the kind of courage that gets applause, but it is courage.

It's not always a matter of getting rid of your RSI completely. You may not be able to do that if you're seriously injured. But, as Australian journalist Theo says, "I have not beaten it. What you do is control and manage it."

Another man talks about "knowing what to do to keep myself working." He says he is no longer "reckless" with his body, which meant typing long, uninterrupted hours at a keyboard. He has changed the way he works, takes care to exercise, and keeps his symptoms under control. He is mindful, he says, of not falling back into what he calls *the hole.*

People who have lived through trauma and learned from it are always more interesting than those who haven't. One woman credits her struggles with RSI with bringing her a newfound serenity. "It's about being realistic about what I take on and trying to deal with things as they come up. I don't spend nearly as much time thinking about work now. I'm much more detached. I'm more centered."

SECONDARY GAINS

One woman was unhappy in her personal life and felt exploited by her job, when she was injured. She has had to fight hard to get what's due her and feels angry all the time. Not surprisingly, she has failed in her attempt at vocational rehabilitation.

Another woman spends hours investigating new therapies and approaches to treatment. Inevitably, however, she finds flaws in whatever new approach she has chosen to try and quickly abandons it. She insists that she knows more than any therapist and that her case is so special and so difficult that few people can treat it. She has been out of work for years and shows no signs of returning.

Yet another woman complains that her arms hurt her so much that she can't cook or clean. She talks about how bad it makes her feel that her sons and husband have had to pick up the slack. When pressed, however, she admits that she likes having their help around the house. She never could get any before she was injured.

All three women are stuck. A mental-health professional would say they are getting *secondary gains* from their injuries. Essentially, a secondary gain is an unconscious gratification a person gains from the injury. It may be avoiding a job you hate, it may be getting attention you want, or it may be myriad other things. Deriving secondary gains does not mean that your pain and disability are not real. Nor is it a problem to enjoy secondary gains for a short period of time. But if you find yourself stuck, unable to progress, consider consulting a mental-health professional. Getting caught up in a secondary gain can prevent you from making a full recovery.

Even if you don't feel stuck, you may want to see a therapist to help understand and cope with the myriad emotions you may be feeling. There are mental-health professionals who specialize in disability and chronic pain. If you don't have insurance or the money to pay for therapy, contact a local mental-health agency. Often, these are run by local charity groups or by local and state governments. They usually will offer fees on a sliding scale, which means what you can afford; and their fees are generally considerably lower than the sliding-scale fees of private therapists. An agency should not turn you away because of an inability to pay.

❧

IS IT ALL IN YOUR HEAD?

A doctor who doesn't understand RSI may fall back on a term to describe your condition: *psychogenic pain.* As explained in chapter 7, that is merely a euphemism for saying that it's all in your head. Of course it's not! But it is a stigma that has long been attached to RSI.

Why? Some people attribute that bias to simple sexism because more women than men are injured. There may be a class bias as well because people in lower-paying office and manufacturing jobs were among the first people to be seriously injured. It may also be because RSI is hard to understand—it's just hard to believe that a seemingly innocuous activity like typing on a computer keyboard, for example, can do so much harm. But remember, nobody thought smoking was a dangerous activity a generation ago, either.

In Australia, where the debate over whether RSI had psychological or physical origins raged during the 1980s, researchers found that people with RSI showed significant disturbances of the nerve pain pathways. The extent of the disturbance of the pain pathways correlated to the patients' own descriptions of their pain. At the same time, psychological tests showed they were not hypochondriacs.

The researchers found that the patients did have higher-than-normal levels of anxiety, depression, anger, and fatigue—but concluded that these emotions were more likely to be the result of the RSI, not the cause. They also found that patients tended to use precise terms to describe their pain— like *throbbing, heavy, exhausting,* and *hot-burning.* That was in sharp contrast to the typically vague terms used by people whose pain was of psychological origin.

Despite the growing scientific evidence that RSI is physical in origin, the stigma persists. Unfortunately, it is often used to blame the victim rather than to find a solution.

✄

DEALING WITH OTHERS

People can be extraordinarily insensitive to the pain and disability of others. With RSI, it's especially difficult because you don't look injured. One woman admitted that she wore splints not only because they seemed to ease her pain but also because they signaled to others that she was injured. Otherwise, she says, people would assume there was nothing wrong.

John, who has had RSI on and off since 1990, says it has been easy to explain his situation to friends and family members, but that it's been harder handling the day-to-day activities that arise as a matter of routine, like "when you're talking to a stranger and they just hand you a package." Or, when he's walking out of a grocery store with a woman, and she's carrying the groceries. "I get a lot of funny looks," he says.

Even when people know there is something wrong, however, they have a hard time knowing how to deal with someone in pain. Some can be supportive and sensitive, others aren't. Remember that you have every right to disregard their opinions. And bear in mind that sometimes their opinions are nothing more than simple prejudice.

Prejudice

Anyone who lives with a disability for any length of time discovers the prejudices many people hold against the disabled. It is so deeply ingrained that few people are aware of it. It is reflected in the consistently patronizing tone of newspaper and television stories about the disabled: They are always about people who have "triumphed" over their physical limitations with extraordinary feats. Rarely is a disabled person covered like any other person in the news—with the same hopes, desires, and fears. The stories about triumph make everyone feel better about disability because they make it seem as if it could not really be as bad as it is. And, of course, if a quadriplegic can be a superathlete, why can't you do the same thing?

Then there are the people who seem to think that having a disability is some sort of character flaw, or that you are somehow "weaker," which is why you got RSI. They treat you as if you have failed in a Darwinian survival race and that your suffering is simply part of the natural order of things. If you try to talk them out of that, you will undoubtedly fail because their conviction is so strong. If you try to point out that it's a prejudice, they won't understand.

It's usually not worth making the effort to get through to such people. Save yourself the heartache, and limit your contact with them as much as possible. Otherwise, you'll undoubtedly hear myriad insensitive comments.

Insensitive Comments

Part of dealing with RSI is handling the thoughtless comments other people make. At one session of an RSI support group, members listed some of the insensitive comments they had heard. With each, nearly everyone in the group laughed in recognition. Here are some of the comments they and others with RSI have mentioned:

"But you don't look like anything's wrong with you."

"It can't really hurt *that* much."

"Isn't there something you can do?"

"We both work on computers. How come I didn't get it?"

"Being on disability must be like being on vacation."

"The company will take care of you. What have you got to worry about?"

"Think about how bad it must be for someone who is really injured."

"At least you've got the time off work."

"Well, if it isn't the gimp!"

"Disabled people work. You don't want to work."

Dealing with such remarks is a personal matter. You may decide to confront the person making the comment, or you may decide just to get out of the conversation. It may depend on how you're feeling at that particular moment, or it may be due to other circumstances. Whatever you choose is up to you. You could try to explain your situation to the person making the comment, but it's not likely to make much difference. Perhaps the best thing to do for your own mental health is to talk about it with someone who understands.

Here are some possible responses to uninvited advice or general comments:

- Explain that you are under a doctor's care and that you prefer to discuss the nature of your injury with your doctor.
- Thank them for their concern, and change the subject.
- Explain that RSI has been well-documented in the medical literature as a real injury and that you can suggest some articles to read—if they are interested.

Dealing with Loved Ones

Pain and disability can also intrude upon intimate relationships. In many ways, it becomes a third party in a relationship. If you are in pain, you're likely to be tired and irritable. A spouse, significant other, or family member may try to be supportive at first but may eventually lose patience. Some may resent having to shoulder more of the work around the home. At the same time, you may feel angry that the people closest to you don't understand what you're experiencing. They have been thrust into new roles that they may or may not want, but so have you.

Or you may have a spouse, significant other, or family member who tries to do everything possible to take care of you. If you, like most people with RSI, are used to taking care of yourself, this can make you feel guilty and uncomfortable. It's hard to watch the people you love shoulder extra burdens while you do nothing. You may worry that the burdens will be so great that you will lose that person.

Sometimes, a loved one will have trouble listening to you talk about your RSI simply because it causes anxiety. It's frightening to see someone you love disabled. It stirs up feelings of loss, abandonment, and one's own mortality. If you find that a loved one is distant, or is unable to listen, you may wrongly assume that that person doesn't care. It may well have more to do with his own fears.

The financial pressures that often accompany RSI can cause additional tension in a relationship. Even if your spouse or significant other doesn't blame you for a loss in income, he is likely to be angry. It is tough to lose income and face the real problems that sometimes go along with that, such as losing a house. Even if you are not at that point, the fear and worry may exist.

Keep in mind that you are not the only one who needs to work through the phases of your loss. The people close to you also need to be allowed to work through the emotional impact of your RSI. You do not live in a vacuum; your life does affect others. RSI can damage—or strengthen—relationships.

There are some ways to try to work it through with your loved ones. First, talk to them. Listen without being judgmental and defensive, and let them express their anger. If you let them know that you understand you are not the only one suffering, they may feel free to talk more openly about the situation. Make the RSI the target of anger and bitterness—not your loved ones.

This is hard to do when you are coping with an injury such as RSI. You may find that you need help. If your injury has caused problems in an important relationship, consider seeing a mental-health professional.

✄
HELPING YOURSELF

There are ways to help yourself ride out RSI's emotional roller coaster. The key is in not allowing yourself to be helpless. Take charge in any way you can. No one will take better care of you than you. Because RSI can be so hard on your self-esteem, in ways that you may not even recognize, it is helpful to find other ways to be productive. Whether it is mastering a mundane task that has confounded you, channeling your energies into a project, or volunteer work that you can physically handle, it helps to find something that enables you to recapture a sense of your own self-worth.

Angela, who has not worked full time since 1992 because her RSI is so disabling, agrees that the psychological toll has been "tremendous." She often feels isolated, anxious and depressed, and has gained fifty pounds. But she tries to look on the positive side. She has joined a church and takes time to explore cultural activities; both give her much joy. And she has purchased a lightweight camera so that she can pursue photography, a longtime interest. For Angela, it is essential "not to focus on your disability twenty-four hours a day" and to do normal things. "I try to keep busy. I try to pursue my interests," she says. "I'm not just sitting here in a heap."

Following are some things that other people with RSI have done. This section is not meant to imply that you should be doing any or all of these things. Concentrating on your recovery may be all you want to do at the moment. These are simply activities that have helped others.

Try Doing Things Differently

If you can find a way to do something you love without hurting yourself, it will give you a sense of mastery. Because of RSI's pain and limitations, it is easy to assume that you won't be able to do any of the things you want to do. The fact is, you can—with help. It may take assistance from a friend or the use of adaptive equipment, but there are ways to get things done. You can cook a meal with adaptive tools, get a headset so you can use the phone, or use a built-up pen to write. Using a buddy system to do chores can be fun. Or it may be even simpler. Perhaps you can continue doing the hobby you love, but do less of it.

It can be frustrating. But you may also find yourself taking pride in your own resourcefulness and creativity. People with RSI often demonstrate extraordinary resourcefulness. And it will certainly improve the quality of your life if you are able to do more. (See chapter 10 for tips on how to do daily tasks.)

Consider Activism

For some people, it helps to be politically involved. In particular, it may be a channel for the anger you feel because of your injury. Advocates of workplace reform say they draw many volunteers from the ranks of the injured; they say they do this work because they don't want what happened to them to happen to others. There are many ways to be politically active that won't hurt your hands: following the issues, joining rallies, giving talks. Knowing that you can make a difference in the lives of others can be immensely satisfying. People who volunteer often say they get more from the experience than they give.

You may find that your interest in activism is temporary, which is fine. Workplace advocates say that people often stop being involved as their own lives get busy with other things. There's nothing wrong with giving what you can and then moving on.

Volunteer or Take a Class

If politics is not to your taste, there are other kinds of volunteer work that doesn't involve using your hands that you might try. Or perhaps there is a class you've always wanted to take. This may be an opportunity to pursue interests you've never had a chance to explore before. Allow yourself to do that, for no other reason than to give yourself a break from the hard work of getting better. Focusing on treatment can be an all-consuming experience; taking a break can help you keep it in perspective.

Get Out of the House

People with RSI often complain about their sense of isolation. It may be due to a lack of understanding among their friends and family, or it may be due to their difficulty in getting around. Some people with RSI can't drive. Others find it difficult to even ride in a car. But if you are feeling homebound, take a walk. Use public transportation. Ask a friend for a ride. It's healthy to get out and partake in the world.

Talk to Others with RSI

Because this injury can be so hard on spouses and family members, it's vital for people with RSI to have a larger support system. For your own mental health, you may want to talk with others who have RSI. They best understand what you're experiencing and often can share ideas with you on how to cope. You may find that you have more to offer to others with RSI than you think.

You can communicate through the informal networks that seem to spring up spontaneously—you get a name from someone, who got a name from someone, etc. Real friendships can form because of these networks. Or you can do it in a more formalized way, through a support group.

For Angela, going to a support group has been key to helping her remain positive. She says her family is not supportive emotionally or financially. "Not having family or friend support is not totally uncommon," she says. You look OK, so it is assumed you aren't ill. Some people are supportive, but it may not be your family or friends—hence the importance of RSI support groups and joining the greater disabled community."

A support group is simply a group of people that shares similar concerns and meets on a regular basis to talk. These people may use the sessions to vent or they may use the sessions to get more information about a particular topic. Typically, support groups try to provide a safe and confidential setting. Usually, there is no fee. Hospitals, nonprofit groups, and labor unions offer sessions for people with RSI across the country. (For a list of some of these support groups, see the appendix.) A support group, run either by a professional or by volunteers, can be an invaluable source of emotional support and information.

If there is no group in your area, one option is to start one yourself. They are really not that much work if you have the right support from a sponsoring organization, and they can be a great way to meet other people and learn more about subjects that interest you. Many support groups invite speakers to cover topics ranging from worker's compensation to treatment options.

One caution: Different people have varying needs for social support, clinical psychologist Hung says. While some people may find a support group immensely helpful, others might find the experience demoralizing. Don't force yourself to participate in one if you don't feel comfortable with it.

Here are some tips on starting a support group:

- *Find a neutral place to meet.* Look for a place that won't charge you, like a church, community center, or non-profit organization. If your doctor or therapist is interested in the idea, he might provide or suggest office space. Avoid meeting in someone's home, since nobody with RSI wants to have to clean house for a session!
- *Enlist support.* If your doctor or therapist is interested, ask for information and ideas. She may not have the time to commit to a support group itself but will likely have helpful suggestions. Or, if you have a friend with RSI who is interested, get him to share the work. That is especially helpful if one of you is unable to attend a particular meeting.
- *Set a regular time for meetings.* It is easiest to keep continuity of the group if you have a regular time and

place. It's easier for everybody to remember. It may also be a good idea to set a time limit for meetings, because that makes it easier for people to plan.

- *Enforce confidentiality.* If people are going to talk about intimate feelings, they need to know that those feelings will be kept confidential. Talking outside the group about what someone might have said will only undermine the entire group.
- *Set ground rules.* These are individual and are up to you and other members. You may decide that everyone attending the group should introduce themselves and take a turn speaking. Or you may want to leave it up to whoever wants to speak. Whatever you decide, it is easier to run a group if you set up ground rules. People will know what to expect and will abide by them.
- *Publicize the group.* Let people know when and where the meetings are. Local newspapers often accept notices of meetings that are open to the public free of charge. Simply write a short notice and send it to the appropriate editor. Call the newsroom to get details on where and to whom to send it. Radio stations and some local television stations will also read notices. You will learn soon enough which media outlets get the most response so you'll be able to target your notices.
- *Set up a contact person or place.* If you are willing to handle phone calls, you can use your own phone as a contact number. If you are meeting in a nonprofit agency or community center, that organization may be willing to field calls for you. Or you can set up a post office box to handle inquiries.
- *Keep it free.* People are far more likely to attend if the support group is free. It's also far less hassle if no money is involved.

Talk to a
Mental-Health Professional

You may find it easier to talk to a mental-health professional one-on-one. There's nothing wrong with that. Don't let embarrassment or shame stop you from getting the help you need. Some disorders, such as anxiety or depression, can grow worse and become a more serious psychological disorder if left untreated, Hung says. With the help of a competent therapist, you will be able to deal more effectively with the problems caused by your injury.

Some people worry that seeing a psychotherapist implies that RSI is all in their heads. The fact is that any kind of illness or injury has an emotional fallout. You wouldn't be human if you didn't have feelings about your condition. Seeing a therapist is merely a way to treat that emotional fallout.

❀
DON'T LOSE HOPE

There is no *right* way to deal with RSI emotionally. Don't beat yourself up for spending what seems like a lot of time in denial or for being depressed. As mentioned earlier, the emotional phases discussed here are normal and are actually a part of the healing process. Each person's path to recovery is unique. Although the path may be rocky, your life will be enriched in unexpected ways because of the experience.

The most important thing you can do for yourself is to remain hopeful. Psychologists who have studied the attitudes of people with chronic injury have found hope to be a powerful predictor of outcome. Simply put, people with high hopes are far better able to persevere in dire circumstances. They suffer less depression, have more mobility, more social contacts, and greater sexual intimacy. They are able to stay involved with life, despite their disability. And they appear to have a higher rate of recovery.

So, keep your hopes high.

CHAPTER 12

NAVIGATING THE FINANCIAL MAZE

Melita has always considered herself an independent, self-sufficient person. She put herself through college and technical school and took pride in the fact that she had worked her way up to a job as a production manager in a company in Minneapolis, where few other women had reached that high a level. After the pains in her hands were diagnosed as carpal tunnel syndrome, she had several surgeries. She tried to return to work, but was too disabled to stay. Melita has been out of work since 1991 and has had to fight "tooth and nail" for benefits. "If I did not have a husband who works and was willing to stick it out," she says, "I would've lost everything."

✄

FINANCIAL
WORRIES

The issue of finances looms large for anyone with RSI. Even if you haven't been forced out of work by RSI, the prospect of being unable to support yourself can be terrifying. RSI often strikes people in the prime of their careers; few ever expected to be disabled, especially by an on-the-job injury. Some people with RSI never thought to buy disability insurance; it's expensive and they didn't think they'd ever need it. Others are reluctant to file for worker's compensation, worried about the stigma attached to it. Without the safety net of disability or worker's compensation, the financial consequences can be significant, sometimes devastating.

Even if you have adequate insurance and employment benefits, you will probably experience some financial losses if you are forced out of work for longer than a few months because disability plans generally do not replace your full salary. In addition, there are other factors that affect your finances: lost pension contributions by your employer and lost opportunity in the form of promotions, raises, and other job opportunities. Even if you manage to stay on the job despite your injury, you may not feel able to pursue other jobs or promotions because of your RSI, or you may not feel that you are seriously considered for them.

Even more frustrating is the fact that the system of benefits—both private and governmental—designed to protect workers often leaves them feeling cheated and abused. This chapter will discuss, in general terms, worker's compensation, disability insurance, and other benefits. Laws vary from state to state, and private policies vary, but there are some general considerations.

WORKER'S COMPENSATION

What is it?

Essentially, worker's compensation is a system of insurance regulated by state governments that reimburses employees for the economic impact of any illness or injury they incur on the job. It is designed to protect employees and employers. It is a no-fault system, which means that you do not have to show that your employer caused the injury; you merely have to show that you were injured on the job. That is not always so easy, and some worker's compensation attorneys argue that it is an adversarial system because a worker's compensation insurance carrier can deny you coverage if it is determined that your injury is not work-related. The burden is on you to prove that your injury is work-related. In addition, if you decide to file for worker's compensation benefits, you waive your right to sue your employer for the injury, except in extreme cases where it can be shown that the employer deliberately intended to harm you.

Worker's compensation has become a hot political issue in recent years as costs have soared and insurers have passed those costs on to businesses in the form of higher premiums. In fact, concerted efforts have been made throughout the United States to limit benefits to workers as a way of lowering costs. Some states, including Illinois, Indiana, and Minnesota, have tried to restrict coverage, specifically of RSI. Lawmakers in Ontario, Canada, have also moved to limit compensation benefits to workers with RSI; and in Australia, RSI has been abolished as a compensable injury.

Attorneys Victor Fusco and Richard Brandenstein, who handle hundreds of worker's compensation cases on Long

Island, New York, say courts have become far less sympathetic to work-related injuries. "It's getting tougher and tougher," Brandenstein says. "Cases we were winning five years ago are getting thrown out today." The attorneys argue that those cases still have merit, but that a more conservative political climate has encouraged the adverse judgments. "They'll always sacrifice the rights of the disabled first," Fusco says.

In addition, they attribute the attitude to an organized effort on the part of insurers to lobby legislators, push news stories about worker's compensation fraud, and pay for ads that cite the high costs of claims. Meanwhile, Fusco and Brandenstein say, workers with real injuries suffer financial losses that should be covered.

Insurers, for their part, claim there is a significant rate of fraud, which will only be fully addressed if it is harder to get benefits. They argue that fraud is driving up costs, which has forced some small businesses to close because owners cannot pay exorbitant worker's compensation premiums. And some insurers argue that RSI is not truly work-related and should not be covered by worker's compensation at all.

The debate won't be resolved anytime soon, but more honest employers do admit that worker's compensation is probably a better deal for employers than for employees because it protects employers from liability lawsuits. As you navigate the insurance maze, understand that a highly charged atmosphere exists, and it has absolutely nothing to do with you or your individual claim.

What's Covered?

Specific benefits vary from state to state, so ask your local worker's compensation board or people in the employment benefits office at your job about exactly what's covered. You are usually better off calling your local board; human resources personnel may not be as well-acquainted with worker's compensation benefits. If you are a member of a union, contact a union representative, although your union representative may not be fully versed in worker's compensation benefits, either. The following are some of the costs that have been covered by worker's compensation:

- Medical costs
- Lost wages, usually two-thirds of your salary, up to a specified cap
- Job retraining
- Prescriptions
- Psychotherapy
- Medical aids, such as splints or TENS machines
- Adaptive devices, such as door handles or driving aids, that are medically prescribed
- Equipment needed to return to work
- Mileage to and from medical appointments

Again, specific coverage varies from state to state. This list is intended to give you an idea of what kinds of questions to ask. Often, if you don't ask, they won't volunteer the information. If worker's compensation doesn't cover certain costs, your disability-insurance plan may.

Patients covered by worker's compensation pay no deductibles and no medical bills. In fact, in some states it is illegal for a doctor or therapist to collect payment directly from a patient covered by worker's compensation.

Who's Eligible?

All states require that employers provide worker's compensation benefits to their employees; so if you work for someone else, you are most likely covered. (Federal employees are covered by a separate law, as are longshoremen, railway workers, coal miners, and sailors.) Employees are not required to pay for those benefits, although some states are pushing for legislation that would require employees to pay premiums for worker's compensations insurance, just as they do for health insurance.

If you are self-employed or work as an independent contractor, you should buy your own policy.

To be eligible for benefits, *you must file a claim*. It is not enough to merely notify your employer. You need to file a written claim.

Dealing with the System

Few people are prepared to take on the worker's compensation bureaucracy. The hardest part is to not take it personally. There is always a feeling that if "they" simply understood, "they" would do the right thing. Unfortunately, the system doesn't always work well. Horror stories about the difficulty of securing benefits abound. Marion, a secretary who required surgeries on both arms, had to wait a year before she got approval for the first surgery. "The worst part was that I was still in pain and I couldn't do anything about the pain," she says. She recalls crying "hysterically" to her worker's compensation lawyer on the phone, saying, "You don't understand, I'm in pain."

There was little he could do to speed up the bureaucracy. The system is slow, impersonal, and often arbitrary. As Vincent

Rosillo, a worker's compensation attorney in New York City, told a conference on RSI, "The pain and suffering you go through is not a component of your worker's compensation case."

Here are some things you can do that will make it easier— though not easy—to receive worker's compensation benefits:

1. *File a claim immediately.*

This can be difficult with RSI because the onset may be gradual, and initially you may not understand its cause. But it is important to file a claim as soon as you know you have a work-related injury. Most states have a statute of limitation on filing claims; it can range from just two days up to thirty. If you don't file a claim within that time period, you will not be entitled to receive benefits, regardless of the extent of your injury.

The other difficulty in filing a claim for RSI is that worker's compensation is geared to accidents, not the gradual development of injury or illness. A form may ask you to write down the date of your accident; with RSI, that can be difficult to pinpoint. If you cannot supply an approximate date, discuss it with your doctor.

You may also feel reluctant to file a claim, fearing it will disrupt your relationship with your employer or that it may attach a stigma to you. Most of the time, it will. But you must protect yourself, and it is illegal for an employer to retaliate against you for filing a worker's compensation claim. That doesn't mean retaliation doesn't occur, and any fears you have may be justified. But you are entitled to the benefits.

2. *Seek medical attention immediately.*

This not only helps establish your claim, but it is essential with an injury such as RSI. The longer you delay treatment, the greater risk you run of experiencing a more severe injury.

In many states you have the right to select your own doctor; however, in some, your employer can choose your doctor or give you a list of doctors you may see. Advocates for injured workers criticize that system because they feel company-approved doctors are less likely to support your claim. If you are in a state where you can choose your own doctor, be prepared for the fact that some physicians won't accept worker's compensation. They dislike the lower fees they are paid for patients covered by worker's compensation, and they hate the extra paperwork. The spread of managed-care plans, however, has forced more and more doctors to accept lower fees and more red tape, so worker's compensation doesn't seem like such a stepchild these days. But there is still a bias, which is particularly unsettling when you are in pain and seeking treatment.

The best advice is to avoid any doctor reluctant to accept worker's compensation. You need a doctor who is willing to be your advocate.

3. *Give your doctor a clear work history.*

This is particularly important with RSI, Fusco and Brandenstein say, because a case will be rejected if your doctor does not file paperwork establishing the work-related nature of the injury. "Someone may tell the doctor, 'I was picking up my kid, and my wrists started to hurt.' The doctor doesn't take down any more [information], and you've got an uphill fight for the next two years," Brandenstein says.

While it may be true that your wrists began to hurt when you were picking up your child, be clear about the work activities you believe caused your injury.

In addition, a doctor reluctant to file a worker's compensation claim may ask that you pay for treatment through private insurance. That may be acceptable to you in the beginning, but if that insurance runs out, it is highly unlikely that worker's compensation will pick up the rest of the tab if further treatment is required.

4. *Be consistent.*

It is important to be consistent in what you tell doctors, therapists, and anyone else you speak to about your RSI. Any inconsistency is likely to be documented in medical records and can be the basis for turning down a claim. It is easy to forget details of your case, especially if you have been dealing with it for a long time. Avoid this by keeping track of what you say and do.

5. *Mention it to coworkers.*

Many people are uncomfortable talking about their RSI to coworkers. If you are comfortable with doing so, mention your injury. Such a conversation could become a part of the evidence establishing your claim to worker's compensation. In one New York case, a woman was denied worker's compensation because she had not mentioned her injury to coworkers, and the judge determined it must not have been serious because she did not feel the need to tell anyone on the job.

6. *Decide whether you want an attorney.*

The worker's compensation system can be confusing and intimidating even for the best and brightest. It is a specialized area of the law, and it is changing. Hearings are brief, the lawyers talk in jargon, and the insurance company is always represented.

The choice is up to you, of course. If your claim is not being challenged by your employer, and if you are comfortable with the vagaries of the law, you may be able to handle it yourself. If your case is being challenged by your employer, you may want to get an attorney. An employer challenging your claim is refusing to pay benefits; an attorney may nonetheless be able to get you benefits. Even if your employer is not inclined to challenge your case, your employer's insurance company may do so and will be represented by an attorney. It is in the insurance company's financial interests to keep the amount of claims down; some challenge worker's compensation claims routinely.

In many states, your lawyer's fees will be paid out of your worker's compensation stipend or out of any eventual settlement, so that you won't have to pay money out of pocket. Generally, lawyers do not charge for an initial consultation on worker's compensation matters. In some states, it's illegal for a lawyer to accept money directly from a claimant.

Those people who think attorneys are an unnecessary expense point out that in some states, lawyers derive the bulk of their fees from lump-sum settlements, which may encourage them to settle certain cases rather than seek continuing payments. Others point out, however, that seeking advice from professionals who know the system can head off problems.

Problems
You May Encounter

Many of the people who've been through the worker's compensation system find it hard to believe that it was designed to protect them. It was, of course, but as with any government bureaucracy, things don't always go smoothly. Nor is the system a forum in which to air your grievances. It is simply a mechanism for paying your medical bills and replacing some lost wages. You may encounter some of the following problems:

Your employer may controvert your case   To controvert your case is to challenge it. Some employers simply have a policy of controverting all worker's compensation claims. For some, it's a way to discourage other employees from filing worker's compensation claims, which can quickly become expensive. For others, it's a matter of demonstrating how cost-conscious they are. It probably isn't a personal matter but rather about the company's bottom line. Sometimes it isn't policy but is because your employer doesn't believe you are injured or that your injury is work-related.

Whether it's personal or a matter of policy doesn't make much difference if you are the one whose case is being controverted. It does mean, however, that you will have to make your case in order to receive benefits. That means establishing a medical record of your injury. If your RSI resulted from an obvious accident on the job, you should ask any witnesses to sign statements. You may also want to get a worker's compensation lawyer because the issues can quickly become complicated.

Some workers have lost their claims for compensation because they filed them after the statute of limitations had expired. Others have lost after their employers were able to raise questions about the causation, linking it instead to outside activities, such as sewing or even fishing. Courts also have ruled in favor of employers who have been able to point to other conditions that have been linked to carpal tunnel syndrome, such as diabetes and obesity.

Sometimes, workers have lost their suits for benefits because the laws in their states are narrowly written. In 1996, the Supreme Court of Virginia ruled that three people with RSI, two chicken processing–plant workers and a copy editor at an advertising firm, were not entitled to worker's compensation simply because RSI was not considered an occupational disease under state law. In a 1997 case, the Supreme Court of Idaho denied worker's compensation benefits to a grocery store meat cutter because he was not completely disabled by his carpal tunnel syndrome. Even though he had to apply hot towels to his hands to relieve the pain so he could continue working, the court found he had not suffered a disabling injury because he had not taken time off work.

The point is that you may be right and justified in seeking worker's compensation benefits, but that's not always enough to get you what you need. You may need help, whether you seek it from a lawyer or a union. You may be able to appeal to a hearing officer or a state agency, or you may have the right to sue. (More on that in chapter 13.)

Expect long delays   The worker's compensation system is literally jammed with people across the country. Hearing officers simply cannot keep up with the demand. It may take a year before you get your first hearing. If your employer has not controverted your claim, you will likely be able to get medical treatment before your hearing. However, if your employer is controverting your claim, you'll have to wait.

This part of the system is particularly maddening for people with RSI. Even if you want to pay your doctor and therapist yourself for your treatment, this is illegal in some states if you have filed a worker's compensation claim. That means you simply have to wait. If you have to appeal your case, it can literally take years. It's not fair, but it's the way the system often works.

Angela, a secretary who developed carpal tunnel syndrome severe enough to warrant surgery on both hands, is still fighting for worker's compensation five years after filing her claim. She has seen delays from her file inadvertently fail to be transcribed and her file being lost to demands for more testimony in her case. "It's been a totally frustrating experience," she says.

She refuses to give up, however. "It's not a huge sum that we're talking about, but, for me, it's the difference between eating and not eating," she says. "Plus, it's the injustice of it." She is barely getting by now because she receives Social Security Disability benefits and because she has savings, but as the time wears on, those savings are dwindling.

The doctor you want won't take worker's compensation As mentioned, some doctors don't accept worker's compensation because of the lower fees and the additional paperwork. In addition, some specialists you might want to see, like a rheumatologist, have little reason to accept worker's compensation because most of the people they see don't have work-related injuries.

Even when your doctor does accept worker's compensation, you may encounter problems. One woman recalls bitterly how difficult it was for her to get appointments with her doctor, a well-known RSI specialist. The office manager kept putting her off, telling her that she had to come in person to make appointments or that she was unable to find the scheduling book to pencil her in. When the woman's husband, who had private insurance (and a different last name), called to make an appointment, he got one the next week. The woman surmised that the office staff simply didn't want to deal with the red tape of worker's compensation. Infuriated by such second-class treatment, she switched doctors.

Some people see receiving worker's compensation as a stigma Like the woman who discovered that her doctor's office staff didn't want to give her an appointment because her case was paid by worker's compensation, many RSI patients have been infected by the stigma associated with it. "A lot of times, people just assume you're faking it," said one woman, "as if you're putting in all this time in treatment for the fun of it!"

In fact, there is little financial incentive to fake a worker's compensation injury because your wage is not replaced in full. Yes, frauds exist everywhere, but any doctor or therapist who has treated people with RSI will tell you that the real problem is getting patients to *stop* working. Usually, they go to great lengths to stay on the job. Andy, a Webmaster in Ann Arbor, Michigan, no longer types with his fingers because it's too painful. Instead, he types using the eraser ends of pencils.

Your records are not as confidential as you think Think carefully about what you disclose to your doctor or therapist. Although they must keep what you tell them confidential, they have to file records in order to get paid. And increasingly, insurers are demanding to know more and more about patients' conditions before they pay. It is a frustrating and difficult line for a health-care provider to walk. Psychotherapists admit to lying occasionally on the forms just to ensure their patients get treatment. That is not to say that you should lie, but you should know that your records are not as private as you might like. Be careful of what you say.

Your paperwork doesn't just disappear into a void. It is handled by any number of people along the way, as well as electronic "switchers," which are data-collection tools embedded in computer software that intermittently sweep records for data collectors. This is a particularly troubling issue for someone who has filed a worker's compensation claim. Some companies actually have compiled databases of workers who have filed worker's compensation claims and sell that information to employers, who use it to screen out what they view as potentially troublesome prospective employees. Surveys of Fortune 500 companies have shown that some 50 percent of the largest companies in the United States receive and use medical data in employment decisions.

The gathering and sale of medical information have become big business for a wide array of companies, and much of it—in fact, virtually all of it—is done without the patient's knowledge or consent. A 1997 study by the prestigious National Research Council called for better controls on medical-records databases. It warned that federal plans to use universal identifiers, such as Social Security numbers, to link all of a patient's records could encourage discrimination in insurance, employment, and credit.

That means you could have difficulty getting health or disability insurance after filing a worker's compensation claim. The insurance industry has a pretty good handle on health information in the United States, primarily because of the Medical Information Bureau. The MIB, as it is known to industry insiders, is a Boston-based consortium of health, life, and disability insurers that maintains for its members a huge database of information on fifteen million Americans.

Insurance companies, which collect health information whenever someone applies for a health, life, or disability policy, provide the information to MIB. Once there, it is stored for seven years. It is used by insurance companies to check on the truthfulness of applicants and to weed out high-risk cases. Consumer advocates say the big problem with MIB information is that it isn't always accurate, in much the same way that information from credit-rating companies is often flawed. And although insurers are not supposed to make final decisions based on MIB information, consumer advocates fear that people might get turned down because of inaccurate information—and never even know it.

You can request your records from MIB. For an eight-dollar fee, the bureau will disclose an individual's records. (See the appendix for further information.)

Insurance companies, by the way, are not entitled to complete access to your medical records, even though many company officials think they are. If, for example, you saw a mental-health professional while in the hospital and did not ask the insurance company to pay the bill for therapy, the company is not entitled to see it. But it is still part of your hospital record. You can protect yourself by signing an authorization only for the records covered by insurance. State that clearly to hospital personnel to make sure that your wishes aren't lost in the shuffle.

Checks may be delayed by your worker's compensation carrier

This happens more often than you might think. Delays, whether deliberate or accidental, are common. Therapists and doctors complain that payment of bills can be delayed for months. Technically, this is not supposed to be your problem, but it can disrupt your relationship with your health-care provider. Most people, no matter how caring, don't want to work without being paid. If you need to get involved in order to continue treatment, call your carrier and explain the problem. Sometimes, a phone call is enough to get things back on track. More often than not, however, it takes more than one phone call.

There may also be miscalculations in what you are owed. Keep careful track of expenses. If you are entitled to mileage reimbursement to and from medical appointments, calculate the amount you are owed yourself. If you are entitled to reimbursement for adaptive devices, submit receipts and keep copies. One woman recalls, "In all the time I was dealing with worker's comp, there were lots of mistakes—and not one of them was in my favor."

Expect an independent medical exam   This is not really a problem because it is routine. It is listed here because some RSI patients find the prospect of an independent medical exam frightening—and even a little offensive. Such an exam is used to check up on you, to make sure you're not faking. Yes, it's offensive to anyone who is suffering a legitimate injury, but it is one of the few ways the system has to protect its investment. As a taxpayer, you should be glad independent exams are conducted.

However, an independent medical exam can be particularly difficult with RSI because many doctors are still not familiar with it. If you are ordered to have an independent medical exam, you must go or you could lose your benefits.

During the exam, keep track of how much time the doctor spends examining you. It could be as little as five minutes. Note the questions asked and tests performed. This information will be important if you need to appeal an adverse decision. This is another instance where your own doctor can go to bat for you by filing a report on your injury. In some states, the worker's compensation system gives more weight to the opinion of the treating doctor.

Be prepared for the possibility of some pain and soreness after an independent medical exam. A doctor unfamiliar with your case will not understand that certain movements and physical tests may cause your symptoms to flare up later.

❈ DISABILITY INSURANCE

Rita, a medical-records transcriptionist who developed severe RSI when she was twenty-nine, never bought long-term disability insurance. "I figured I was young, that I wouldn't need it, and I didn't like the policy my company was offering," she says. "Who knew?"

She has been out of work for seven years, receiving only a small worker's compensation check. She feels lucky because her husband and family have been supportive, but she is also chagrined that she has had to rely on her parents financially.

"That's pretty tough at my age," she says.

Rita's story is not uncommon. Many people eschew buying disability insurance for a variety of reasons. Some occupations can't get it. If you don't have it, buy it if you can. Even if you do have it, there are some things you should know about your rights. There are many types of disability insurance, but they basically fall into two categories: short-term and long-term.

Short-Term Disability

Some states require employers to provide short-term disability benefits to employees who are disabled. The amount and duration of benefits vary and may depend, in part, on the number of years you've been with your company. You need to ask your employment benefits office what you have to do to get short-term disability benefits if you have to go out of work as a result of your RSI. You can also buy private short-term disability insurance.

Typically, the paperwork is less involved for the employee on short-term disability. You may need only a few weeks of rest before being able to return to work. In some cases, you may be able to get short-term disability for up to six months, until long-term disability kicks in. Again, the duration varies, but the maximum amount of time covered by short-term disability benefits is typically six months.

Long-Term Disability

There are various long-term disability policies available to consumers. If you work for someone else, you may have as one of your employee benefits the chance to buy disability insurance through your company. The advantage of that is that you are likely to get a cheaper rate. The disadvantage is that you have no choice about the kind of policy you buy. Some employers provide disability insurance at no cost to the employees. If disability insurance is provided by your employer, the benefits are taxable.

The other option is to buy it privately. If you do that, it is likely to be more expensive, but you'll have more freedom of choice. If you buy your own policy, the benefits are not taxable. Everyone should buy disability insurance. No one, particularly young people starting their careers, expects to become disabled. But life surprises all of us, which is why the insurance industry does a booming business.

Most policies replace about half of your income, although some will replace up to 80 percent. Insurers are reluctant to replace your entire income because they want to give you a monetary incentive to return to work. Generally, the more reasonably priced policies replace 50 to 60 percent of your salary. You can decide on how much you need by taking stock of your own financial situation. Add up the benefits that you would be entitled to without private insurance, plus your personal resources. Then look at your fixed expenses. That should give you an idea of how much coverage you need.

Two-Year Clause

Exactly what your policy covers probably wasn't entirely clear to you when you bought it. Brochures and promotional literature don't always clearly define disability. Many policies make a small distinction that can make a big difference if you are out of work for a long period of time. That distinction is that they will cover you for up to two years if you are disabled from your *own* occupation; after that, you must be disabled from *any* occupation in order to continue receiving benefits. It's worth finding out if your policy has such a clause.

For example, if a surgeon injured her hand and was unable to perform surgery, she would *not* be covered if her policy defined disability as being unable to do any kind of work. If she could teach or consult, she would not be covered. But, if she had a policy that defined disability as being unable to perform her own occupation—surgery—she would be covered.

Other policies will cover you for disability from any occupation indefinitely, although they are probably a little more expensive. Still others will pay you a partial benefit if you can still work but cannot earn as much as you did before. Decide what's best for you.

Other Considerations

Find out whether benefits are adjusted for inflation, if Social Security and worker's compensation benefits are deducted, and how income is defined.

As a consumer, you have the right to see your policy. This may seem obvious, but companies don't always give employees copies of entire policies; instead, they pass out descriptive brochures and other information. But if you have questions about what is covered by your policy, insist on seeing a copy of it. By law, your employment benefits counselor is required to show it to you. You may not discover any surprises, but it can be useful.

Another source of long-term disability insurance may be a fraternal, charitable, or professional organization of which you are a member. Many such organizations provide disability insurance free of charge or at a lower rate to members. You may be entitled to it and may not even know it. Ask. Unions often offer disability pensions or emergency loans for members in need. Again, ask.

Some disability policies will pay for retraining you for another line of work if you are no longer able to do your job. That retraining may include schooling, materials, and moving expenses. Some policies also pay for equipment that enables you to resume working. It's cheaper for a company to have you work rather than to continue paying disability benefits.

One reason many people don't buy disability insurance is that it is so expensive. You can do some comparison shopping by getting quotes from several different companies. *Consumer Reports* occasionally rates the various policies; check your local library for a relevant issue. You will probably get a much more affordable rate if you can buy long-term disability through your employer. If you do that, however, you will have fewer choices in the plans offered, and any benefits you receive are taxable. If you buy long-term disability insurance privately, the benefits are not taxable.

Probably the most important feature in a long-term disability policy is that it be noncancelable by the insurance company. That means you have a guaranteed right to renew it every year and that the insurance company cannot change your benefits. Some holders of cancelable long-term disability policies have been stunned to learn that the benefits they thought they were paying for are no longer available.

If You Have Your Own Business

As a business owner, it is especially important to buy disability insurance and maintain good records. It is also essential to have good overall insurance coverage. If you have an overall business-owner's policy, it may not cover an assistant who is working for you but not on the payroll, because you decided the paperwork was not worth it. Most insurance policies require that employers carry worker's compensation insurance for anyone who works for you on a regular basis. If your assistant is injured while working for you, your business-owner's policy may not cover it. Be sure to check before anything happens.

Disability Insurance
Checklist

In summary, here is a list of questions you should ask when buying a disability policy:

- What percentage of my income is paid out as benefits?
- How is income defined? (This may be an important question for those whose income includes overtime or commissions.)
- How long is the coverage? (Cheaper policies cover two to five years of disability.)
- How is disability defined?
- Does the policy provide partial benefits if I can still work but not earn my previous income?
- Are benefits adjusted for inflation? If not, can I buy a rider?
- Is it noncancelable?
- Are Social Security Disability and/or worker's compensation benefits deducted?

You may want to talk to a financial planner before purchasing disability insurance to get a better handle on your expenses and determine exactly how much you'll need to cover your expenses if you do become disabled. Because buying disability insurance is an expensive proposition, be realistic about your needs. (For more information on disability insurance, see the appendix.)

Problems You May Encounter

Like worker's compensation, receiving disability insurance benefits to which you are entitled poses its share of problems. It seems ironic that it might be difficult to get or continue to get benefits, especially if you have purchased the policy for your own protection. But disability insurers are as mindful of the bottom line as any other industry and do what they can to reduce costs.

There's a stigma attached to receiving disability   As with worker's compensation, people tend to view people on disability as if there is something wrong with them. They may think they're malingering, or they may think they're simply crazy. It's particularly hard with RSI, sufferers say, because you rarely look sick or injured.

There's little you can do about that except to keep in mind that you purchased disability as a safety net. Many people buy it and never use it; you just happened to use it. That's good for you and not so good for the insurance company.

You will be pressured to return to work   At some point, your disability insurer is likely to make inquiries about when you plan to return to work. Sometimes the pressure is subtle and intended to help you. Some companies pay for vocational rehabilitation, and their counselors are genuinely interested in helping you.

Other times, the pressure is less subtle. You may find a private investigator knocking on your door one day, unannounced.

It's the company's way of checking up on you, to make sure you're not doing another business on the side while receiving benefits. You are under no obligation to talk to the investigator. If you have a lawyer, tell the investigator that you would be happy to answer any questions in the presence of your lawyer. The investigator's questions may seem innocuous—remember, the best investigators *seem* friendly and innocuous—but you may say something that could damage your case. Most people want to be cooperative, but lawyers advise strongly against that in this instance. Be polite and professional, and limit any conversation until you can talk to your lawyer.

You may have trouble getting a disability policy in the future
Some disability policies terminate when you terminate employment. If you try to buy another disability insurance policy after getting a new job, you may have trouble if you've received benefits before. Although medical records are supposed to be confidential, insurance companies do check huge databases to verify information on potential customers, as well as weed out fraud. If you do not disclose a condition that could have a bearing on the company's decision to issue you a policy, the company can cancel a policy if it finds out.

You may still be able to buy another disability policy, but one that has a rider exempting RSI from coverage. Or you may have to pay a much higher premium to get the coverage you need.

⚘

OTHER BENEFITS

You may be entitled to certain governmental benefits in addition to any other benefits you might receive, for example, if you are a veteran. Ask. The three types of benefits most likely to apply here are Social Security Disability, Medicare, and unemployment benefits.

Social Security Disability

Social Security Disability provides cash and medical benefits to people who can demonstrate that they have been disabled and unable to engage in substantial gainful activity for at least twelve months, or where it appears that a person will not be able to work at all for twelve continuous months. If you apply before you can show you have been disabled for twelve months, you will be turned down.

The system requires clear medical proof that you are disabled. Your medical records are examined, and your age, education, and work experience are reviewed. It is not uncommon to be turned down. It is not enough to be unable to do your own job; you must be unable to do *any* gainful work. It is immaterial whether work exists in your area, a specific job vacancy exists, or you would be hired if you applied for work.

If you are awarded Social Security Disability, there is a waiting period of five months from the time you first became disabled. It can be longer than that because there is a huge backlog in the system. The amount of money you are entitled to depends on your salary and the length of time you've worked. Benefits are payable until you return to work or demonstrate medical improvement. In most cases, you receive Social Security Disability benefits in addition to any worker's compensation benefits, as long as the combined benefits do not exceed 80 percent of your average earnings before the onset of disability. If payments do exceed 80 percent of earnings, a reduction—or offset—is made in Social Security Disability payments. Different factors are used to determine whether there will be an offset and how much it will be. Private pensions and private insurance benefits are not considered in determining the offset.

However, many private disability policies offset Social Security Disability benefits. That means the amount you receive from Social Security Disability is deducted from the amount you are paid. In fact, some disability insurance companies require that their claimants apply for Social Security Disability for just this reason and even hire law firms to help claimants through the application process.

If you decide to apply, you should know that the government worker helping you to fill out your paperwork also takes notes on whether or not you appear disabled, attorneys Fusco and Brandenstein say. You may not even be aware of such note-taking and those notes can become evidence later in a case.

If you are turned down by Social Security Disability, you have the right to appeal within sixty days. Social Security Disability is regarded as difficult to get; most people who apply are turned down initially. However, many win on appeal. The appeals process can be long and complicated, and the outcome is by no means certain, but it may be worth your while. Talk to a lawyer. If you don't know where to find one who specializes in this area of law, call the National Organization of Social Security Claimants Representatives. (See appendix for the phone number.)

Benefits are not paid to someone who continues to have a disabling impairment but engages in substantial gainful work. Nor are they paid to someone who has refused, without good cause, to accept vocational rehabilitation services. Benefits can be terminated if it is determined that you are no longer disabled.

Medicare

Medicare is a federal health-insurance program for people sixty-five and older and for those with disabilities. People with disabilities are defined as people receiving Social Security Disability. You are automatically eligible for Medicare if you have been receiving Social Security Disability for twenty-four months. It is free, but you must pay for deductibles and coinsurance.

Medicare covers some assistive technology, but it must be primarily for medical reasons and must be appropriate for use in the home.

Unemployment Benefits

If you have been terminated from your job, consider applying for unemployment benefits. These are limited in amount and duration, but they could be the safety net you need. To qualify for unemployment benefits, you must be able to demonstrate "recent substantial attachment to the labor market," which means you must show that you were employed for more than a short period of time. You must also be able to show that you are out of work through no fault of your own, and you must be ready and willing to work. That means you can prove that you are actively seeking employment.

You will be ineligible for benefits if you left your job without good cause, were dismissed for job-related misconduct, or capriciously refused to accept suitable employment. You may also be ineligible if you are not completely unemployed: If you are doing part-time or free-lance work, you are likely to be turned down for unemployment benefits. If you are receiving vacation or holiday pay, you may also be ruled ineligible.

Check the rules and filing requirements in your area. Your employer should be able to provide you information, or you can contact your local labor department.

✕

A FINAL WORD

This chapter has provided you with brief, general summaries of the benefits to which you may be entitled. For more detail, check with your employer, union, insurance company, and/or worker's compensation office. Even if your case has not been challenged by your employer or insurer, it makes sense to find out what your benefits are because you could be overlooking something. Human resources personnel often deal with myriad issues and may not always be aware of what's available. Or there may be a clause in an insurance policy that you've never bothered to read. It doesn't hurt to ask.

CHAPTER 13

PROTECTING YOUR RIGHTS

✤

Tim, who describes himself as a "high-performance achiever," was twenty-nine when he was injured in his job as a university librarian in Philadelphia. Also a graduate student at the time, "I was banking a lot on that job to be my springboard," he says. One day, while retyping a midterm paper that he had lost in a computer crash, he hit a "flashpoint" of pain, with hot, numb pains in the center of his palm, as well as shooting pains in his fingers. His shoulders were exhausted, and he felt an overwhelming "whole body" fatigue.

He went to student health services, where he was tested for AIDS. Then, he saw a doctor who himself had suffered carpal tunnel syndrome while in medical school; the doctor immediately recognized Tim's injury. He diagnosed Tim with carpal tunnel syndrome, which was later refined to tenosynovitis and cubital tunnel

*syndrome by a rheumatologist. The physician gave Tim
a splint and told him to go on light duty at work.*

*Tim then went to see his human resources super-
visor. He was stunned when she tried to tell him his
injury wasn't work-related. "I went to her in good
faith. Here I was, a person in pain, trying to find out
how to reduce the pain, and she was like, 'It's not my
fault.'" He says she had advised others with RSI not to
file worker's compensation because "it would all be
paid," but he learned that some of their bills were not
paid by their own health insurance. He made a point
of filing worker's compensation with his employer's
risk-management office, an experience he describes
aptly as "a whole new world." The human resources
supervisor advised him to seek other work.*

*Angered by her threat, Tim researched both RSI
and the law. He was able to preserve his rights, but it
took some tenacity. He has since taken a different job,
where he has been able to get ergonomic equipment.*

⚹

EDUCATE YOURSELF

In protecting your rights, your best weapon is information.
Learn what your rights are, what the laws in your particular
area say, and what your company policy is. You cannot sit back
and expect people to do the right thing. Sometimes they will;
sometimes they won't. If you know what you are entitled to,
you are far more likely to get it. Most people with RSI don't
want to take the time to learn about benefits systems or laws
affecting workers; they're usually busy enough with their own
treatment. Unfortunately, while it may seem like a lot of extra
work, it's often necessary.

"They have to be suspicious of the system," says worker's compensation attorney Richard Brandenstein. "The 'good hands' people are not there."

Some unions and worker advocacy groups periodically offer workshops on worker's compensation, disability, and the law. (See the appendix for some groups.) Check your library for books or magazine articles on the subject, as well as the Internet, which has some detailed information specific to different states. Or, call an attorney and ask whether he offers a free initial consultation. Attorneys Fusco and Brandenstein say they typically spend forty-five minutes with a new client, and about five minutes deciding whether the case is viable; the rest of the time is devoted to explaining how the system works to clear up any confusion and to ease fears. "Once people understand where they're going, they feel better," Brandenstein says.

Armed with a little knowledge, you'll be better able to keep track of your own case, even if you have an attorney. You'll save time and headaches if you know the case's status. You may also find that you have to take other steps to protect yourself, such as filing a grievance with a union or state regulatory agency or filing a lawsuit. This chapter will discuss those options in detail.

Staying on Top of the System

Getting the benefits you need and deserve can be a frustrating and infuriating experience, regardless of the system you are dealing with. Here are some tips:

Keep track of everything   The amount of paperwork generated by a worker's compensation case or a disability case can be staggering. Keep all of it. You never know when you'll need to refer to it. It's helpful to be able to refer to a check number when talking to a representative of an insurance company. It's a way they use to track information, and it's good to let the company know that you, too, are keeping track of things. They don't want to hear about your pain and suffering. They want to process the paperwork.

The most important paperwork you need is that provided by your doctor. She must fill out a form that specifies the diagnosis, whether it is work-related, how it is work-related, other relevant clinical findings, and her signature. Get copies of the important forms; you never know when you might be called upon to supply documentation.

If your case is prolonged or more complicated, you may need to supply other documentation to the Worker's Compensation Board in order to receive benefits. Save stubs of worker's compensation checks, calendars with notes of medical appointments, and copies of prescriptions and medical forms.

Over time, your memory of when certain events occurred may be fuzzy. RSI can be a long-term injury, and it's unlikely that you'll be able to remember each important date. Avoid problems by using your records to keep track of significant events. Those records may become important in the event that you decide to file a lawsuit.

When you fill out forms, fill them out accurately (if there is an error, that can be the basis for an insurance company or worker's compensation board for rejecting a claim), and provide only the information requested. Sometimes, extra details can be misinterpreted and could hurt your claim. Keep it straightforward and simple. If you don't understand something on the form, ask what it means.

If you are worried about being mistreated on the job because of your RSI, take note of comments and incidents that you feel may be discriminatory or related to your RSI. Note the time and place, and briefly describe what happened. Some people keep a diary. That's difficult to do if your pain precludes your ability to write. If that's the case, use a tape recorder to keep the diary. You may never need it, but it will be invaluable if you do. Remember, it is illegal for an employer to retaliate against you for filing a worker's compensation claim.

Be professional and polite Although you may be so angry that you want to scream at your insurance carrier, you are more likely to get results if you are professional and polite. Nobody likes to be yelled at, and people are more likely to help you if they like you.

Sometimes, however, you must be firm and ask to talk to the supervisor if you aren't getting the results you want. In that case, ask for names and addresses. Keep notes of conversations, and let the person on the other end of the line know that you are doing so. (If you cannot write, you can tape the conversation. Some states require that you ask permission to do so, others do not.) People are less likely to brush you off if they think you are going to create a problem for them.

Don't let anyone pressure you into returning to work before you're ready Most RSI patients who have been forced out of work by their injury want to return to work as soon as possible. Add to that calls from employers asking when you're going to return, as well as pressure from a disability insurance company seeking to stop paying benefits, and you could feel overwhelmed. But going back to work too soon can cause you more pain and injury. Before making that decision, talk it over carefully with your doctor. Reinjury can be a devastating experience physically and emotionally. Don't take chances with your health.

Don't take it personally It is difficult not to take it personally when your financial security is threatened. But the fact is, the system doesn't care about your personal integrity, your needs, or the unfairness of what has happened to you. It requires demonstrable proof of a disability, and the standards of proof vary. They may not always be fair. Try to set aside your feelings about it, and follow the rules set up by the system. If you can, you will have a much greater chance of success.

Don't give up The delays and insults that occur can wear you down and make you want to throw in the towel. Don't. Regard getting your benefits as part of your job. Be persistent. If you prevail, the satisfaction you'll feel will be well worth the effort.

Sometimes, despite your best efforts, your rights will be violated. If that's the case, you may be able to sue for monetary damages or file a complaint with a regulatory agency.

IF YOUR RIGHTS HAVE BEEN VIOLATED

If you have been injured on the job, your basic right to personal safety in the workplace has been violated—but that may not matter in a court of law or even to a state regulatory agency. You may have a cause for action, such as a grievance, formal complaint, or lawsuit, depending on the circumstances of your case and the laws in your area. First, determine if you have a specific cause for action. Here are some questions to ask:

- Has your insurer failed to reimburse you for medical costs in a timely manner or as spelled out in your policy?
- Has your insurer failed to provide you with a full copy of your policy specifying your benefits?
- Has your company denied you equal job benefits or treated you differently from other employees because of your RSI?

- Have you asked your employer to make reasonable accommodations that would allow you to continue
working, and has he refused to make such accommodations?
- Has your employer limited your opportunities at work
because of your RSI (in a way that you can document)?
- Has your employer failed to provide a safe working environment?

These are just a few of the situations that people face. If
you answered yes to any of these questions, you may have a
cause for action.

There are some instances in which you may feel your
rights have been violated, but legally, they have not. For example, an employer has the legal right to refuse to pay your medical bills until your claim is approved by the state worker's
compensation system. Such a scenario is frequently encountered by people with RSI; it's infuriating and frustrating but
not illegal. (In fact, it makes sense.) Or a disability insurer may
send a private detective to check up on you. This may be offensive, but it's not illegal.

To fight back, focus on the facts. Set aside your personal
feelings about the unfairness of the situation. It is unfair, but
you are more likely to get results if you have a basic understanding of your legal rights. You don't have to become a
lawyer, though you may need to consult one. (Many attorneys
offer a free initial consultation.)

Dealing with Insurance Companies

When an insurance company sells you a policy, whether it's
health insurance or disability insurance, it is obligated to abide
by the contract you sign at purchase. That means it must pay

the benefits it says it will, in the time period specified. To save money, some insurance companies may delay payment. That may achieve cost-flow savings for them, but it can be devastating to someone dependent on the checks. If you have a problem, call the company. That is your right. (Use the company's 800 number if it has one—and most do—there is no reason you should foot the bill for the call.)

In addition, insurance-company representatives are not allowed to make discriminatory or derogatory statements to policyholders. If that has happened to you, take note of it. Immediately, ask to speak to the person's supervisor and report the incident. Get names. You want it on record as soon as possible. Let them know that you will not tolerate such behavior.

If a phone call doesn't get results, write a letter. If you cannot write because of your injury, dictate it to a sympathetic friend or family member. Send it certified mail, return-receipt requested, so that the insurance company cannot claim it never received your complaint. Ask for a response in writing.

If you feel that your insurance company has not been treating you fairly, complain to the regulatory agency in your state, usually the state insurance department, which oversees insurance. Because insurance companies perform a fiduciary function—that is, they take in money under the terms of legal contracts—they are regulated by the states in which they do business. Several states, including New York, Pennsylvania, and California, have particularly strict, consumer-oriented insurance laws. Sometimes the simple threat of a complaint to a regulatory agency is enough to get what you want. If you cannot find the number of your state insurance department, you can try contacting the National Association of Insurance Commissioners for the listing of your local department. When you call the state insurance department, ask for the consumer section.

If you need to go further, you might want to contact an attorney. You could also try contacting the National Insurance

Consumers Organization. (For address and phone information, see the appendix.) This organization cannot represent you, but its staff may be able to offer advice or refer you to someone who can help you.

Dealing with Your Employer

Advising anyone on how to deal with an employer is difficult because individual relationships vary. But remember, no matter how good your relationship is with your employer, it can quickly become strained if you are deemed as costing the company money. Again, it's important to try to set aside personal feelings—which can be difficult to do—and to try to figure out the best way to get what you need.

Any reputable lawyer will tell you that your first step should be to try to work it out with your employer. That can be hard, especially if your employer is unsympathetic (although, people often make unfair assumptions about what their supervisors will do in any given situation). Here are some suggestions on dealing with your employer.

Approach your employer in a calm and professional manner
Don't rail about the injustice you have suffered. You *have* suffered an injustice, but you are less likely to get what you want if you ram that fact down your employer's throat. It's ridiculous, but many people expect injured workers not to be angry about their situation. You have every right to be angry, but this is not the place to let it show. It is appropriate, however, to be firm and assertive.

Explain your situation   Your employer may not understand what RSI is and you may have to educate her. Don't expect your employer to grasp the concept immediately. Even if your employer doesn't understand your situation, you have fulfilled your obligation by explaining it.

State what you need specifically   It's much easier for an employer to deal with a specific request rather than generalities. Say, for example, that you need a wrist rest for your computer keyboard or a headset for your telephone. It is reasonable to ask for these items, and it is reasonable to expect an employer to supply them. (More on this point will be discussed in the section in this chapter on the Americans With Disabilities Act.)

Rely on your doctor   If your doctor feels you must take time off from work because of your RSI, have her write a note, and present it to your employer. The company is likely to be far more responsive if it is presented as medical advice.

Don't threaten   Even if you feel your rights have been violated, a threat generally won't get you too far. If you do make a threat, be prepared to follow through with it.

Suggest solutions   Sometimes the help you need may not even cost the company any money. It may be a matter of reassigning tasks that are harmful to you and allowing you to take on other work. A reasonable employer will be relieved if you come up with a solution that's workable and will respect you for offering one.

If you don't get the results you want, you may have to explore other channels. For example, if you are a member of a union, talk to your union representative. Find out if there is a management-employee safety committee. This is a perfect forum for an RSI grievance. If that doesn't work, you may have to file a formal grievance against the company. Your union can advise you on how.

If You're Fired

Sometimes, negotiation doesn't work. People with RSI have been fired from their jobs after taking time off for their injuries. Although you should not be fired solely because you filed a worker's compensation claim, you are not immune from being terminated or laid off while you are out on leave. Check your company policy or employee contract for the exact wording of your employer's policy on worker's compensation. There may be language that is helpful to you.

If your company has at least fifty employees, it is covered by the federal Family and Medical Leave Act, which permits eligible employees up to twelve weeks of unpaid leave for family and/or medical reasons. Even if you are out on worker's compensation, you may be covered by that law. Consult an attorney.

You may also be covered under the Americans with Disabilities Act, which applies to companies with at least fifteen employees. Under some circumstances, being fired could be considered discriminatory. The law does not protect you against general layoffs. The key here is that a disabled employee may not be treated differently from any other employee as long as he can perform the essential functions of his job. (The ADA will be discussed in greater depth later in this chapter.) Again, consult an attorney.

✷
FILING SUIT

If all else fails, you may consider filing suit. Check your employment contract. More and more companies are requiring employees to sign a consent form agreeing to take disputes to arbitration, rather than court. Often, signing away your right to sue is a condition of employment, and you may not be fully aware of the implications of doing so. Although several cases have challenged such agreements, courts generally have upheld them. Advocates of mandatory arbitration argue that it is a fair way to resolve disputes without the expense of a trial. Opponents argue that it strips workers of their right to a day in court.

Federal workers seeking to retain lawyers are also treated a little differently. Unlike employees of private companies who can get their legal fees paid through contingency plans, federal workers do not have that option. Federal workers cannot sue their employer—the government—because it is immune from suit. And in one 1997 case, a U.S. District judge in Maryland ruled that postal workers could not sue the company that made a letter-sorting machine they claimed caused their RSI because the company was a government contractor and therefore immune from lawsuits.

If you think you have grounds for a lawsuit but are afraid you cannot afford an attorney, there are legal referral services for the disabled that can put you in touch with a lawyer who will give you an initial consultation at little or no cost. Call your local bar association to see if it provides such a service.

People with RSI who have filed suit have typically filed three types: worker's compensation, product liability, and discrimination.

Worker's Compensation Lawsuits

Injured workers in the United States and Europe have filed suit to win worker's compensation benefits for RSI. Their success has been uneven, depending on the laws in their areas. In general, plaintiffs have had more success when the work-related nature of the injury is well established, and they've had less success when the onset of the injury has been gradual and could have been attributed to other factors. One bitter RSI sufferer, who won her worker's compensation case after seven years of fighting, says, "It's easier to prove a murder case."

In one 1996 worker's compensation lawsuit, a Maryland autoworker developed carpal tunnel syndrome in both hands and received partial benefits based on the determination that he had lost 15 percent use of his hands. After several unsuccessful surgeries and a period of time on light duty, he was reassigned to assembly-line work; his symptoms flared up, and he was urged not to return to work. He filed a new compensation claim for full benefits, citing his continued exposure to a hazardous workplace. The State Appeals Court acknowledged that the reassignment probably exacerbated his symptoms, but ruled that under the law he was not entitled to worker's compensation.

Product-Liability Lawsuits

Other injured workers have filed suit against the manufacturers of the electronic equipment—from computer keyboards to price scanners—they claim injured them. The suits have been based on two legal premises: that the manufacturers failed to provide a safe piece of equipment; and that they failed to warn the users of possible risks or defects of the equipment. To date, plaintiffs have had little success. Most keyboard cases that have gone to trial have resulted in defense verdicts, while other cases have been dismissed before trial. Product-liability attorneys say the political climate is increasingly hostile to such suits, and they point to efforts by the U.S. Congress to cap or do away with damage awards in such cases.

Product-liability suits are difficult to win, which is why some lawyers are reluctant to handle such suits. They want what lawyers consider a "clean" plaintiff, someone who doesn't have other medical factors that might have contributed to her injury or other technical legal problems, as well as a clear case of loss resulting from the injury caused by the product. Such suits also often require much time and the expense of hiring experts to testify.

In the case of keyboard litigation, one recent ruling changed the standard on expert testimony, effectively prohibiting many of the experts whom plaintiffs' lawyers had planned to call. In addition, manufacturers can come up with a variety of defenses: Workers misused their product, failed to follow directions, or knew the product was dangerous but continued to use it anyway.

In 1995, an Eagan, Minnesota, woman lost a closely watched case against IBM. She had sued the company, claiming she had suffered permanent RSI after working on an IBM computer while working at Eagan High School. The jury did not believe the plaintiff had any injury and was not persuaded that any design defect existed in the keyboard. The woman also sued Apple Computer and settled with the company for an undisclosed sum.

In December 1996, the first successful RSI suit against a computer company was widely reported. A jury awarded almost six million dollars to three New York-area women who worked for different companies but on the same equipment for injuries related to computer keyboard use. The defendant, Digital Equipment Corp., had failed to warn customers even after being fined by the Occupational Safety and Health Administration in 1989, according to the plaintiffs' attorney. Two of the women suffered from carpal tunnel syndrome and the third from cubital tunnel syndrome. Then in May 1997, a federal judge threw out the verdict, saying a medical report appeared to indicate that one plaintiff's injury was not work-related. He ordered a new trial.

One result of the RSI product-liability litigation is that several major computer manufacturers, like Compaq Computer Corporation and NEC Corporation, have placed warning labels on their equipment. In addition, alternative keyboards have gained a stronger foothold in the marketplace. Microsoft's "natural" keyboard, for example, has a banked design believed to be easier on the hands and wrists. Even so, the company has placed a warning on it and offers on-line advice on typing and posture.

If you do decide to file a product-liability suit and can find a lawyer willing to take you as a client, you will likely be charged a contingency fee, which is a percentage of any damages you receive if you win the case. That means you don't pay for the lawyer's time. The fee could be one-third of any damages awarded; in some states, it is set by the judge. Or you may be able to negotiate your fee with the lawyer. Some may charge you expenses as they go along; others will add it to their contingency fee if you win the case. If you lose, you may be obligated to pay the lawyer's expenses. Those can add up quickly.

The amount of damages that might be collected in such a suit varies. It depends on the extent of the injury, age, income level prior to injury, and ability to work. Most product-liability suits are settled out of court because trials are costly for both sides.

The statute of limitations for filing such a suit varies from state to state, but it is usually two to three years. Some states have moved to discourage product-liability lawsuits by placing caps on awards and limiting the fees attorneys can charge. This issue also has been a subject of debate in the U.S. Congress, as manufacturers have complained of high awards and frivolous suits. In fact, awards in product-liability suits have often been reduced or overturned on appeal, although those reductions are rarely widely reported.

Americans With Disabilities Lawsuits

The third type of suit possible for disabled workers is allowed under the 1990 Americans With Disabilities Act (ADA). Although the law is still relatively new, scores of people—including those with RSI—have filed suits under it. If you meet certain standards set by the ADA, you may be eligible to file suit as well.

✂

AMERICANS WITH DISABILITIES ACT (ADA)

What Does the Law Say?

The Americans With Disabilities Act is generally considered a well-written law. It bars discrimination against disabled people in hiring, promotion, and other conditions of employment. It also requires an employer to make "reasonable accommodations" for disabled employees, unless that accommodation would cause an "undue hardship." Finally, it prohibits retaliation against employees who exercise their rights under the ADA.

Much has been written about what constitutes a reasonable accommodation. Most surveys of accommodations show that the majority is inexpensive, or cost nothing at all. A University of Iowa study of Sears, the third-largest retailer in the United States, found, for example, that accommodations for employees with carpal tunnel syndrome, shoulder injury, and limited arm use cost nothing. The company limited hours, rotated jobs, provided rest periods, and offered temporary light-work duty.

Examples of accommodations that the ADA would include:

- Restructuring a job so that marginal functions are done by someone else.
- Reassigning the disabled employee to a vacant position (the company is not required to create a new position).
- Modifying a work schedule.
- Offering light duty.
- Providing special equipment.
- Providing readers or interpreters (which might be interpreted to include transcribers, for people with RSI).

Some examples of specific accommodations employers have provided under the ADA include arranging for someone who cannot drive to take public transportation or work at home; allowing an employee with poor physical stamina to take more rest breaks; and allowing an employee to shift his schedule by two hours twice a month to accommodate medical appointments. For ideas on what kind of accommodation might work for you, call the Job Accommodation Network for free information. (See the appendix for the phone and address.)

Whether any of these accommodations force an undue hardship on the employer is decided on a case-by-case basis.

Who Is Covered?

The Americans With Disabilities Act is designed to protect qualified disabled workers. To be considered disabled under the law, you must have a permanent physical or mental impairment that limits one or more major life activities. Examples of major life activities include caring for oneself, working, doing manual tasks, and lifting and reaching. If a person is unable to do a single, particular job, he may not be considered disabled. Or, if the disability is deemed temporary because it can be treated with surgery or some other intervention, the person is not likely to be considered disabled.

If you have a chronic, disabling condition that is permanent but under control, you are still protected by the ADA. One example is a diabetic who takes insulin. RSI might also be considered such a disability, depending on the circumstances of the case.

A disabled person is covered by the ADA only if she is deemed qualified. That means an employee must be able to perform the essential functions of the job, with or without accommodation. If the employee is unable to do that, he is not covered. However, if you were working in the job when you were injured, it is likely the employer deemed you competent to perform the essential job functions. If typing is an essential function of your job, and you can still do it with an alternative keyboard or a voice-activated computer, you would probably be deemed qualified.

Case law pertaining to RSI on this point is sketchy, but several court decisions in the 1990s have rejected the notion that carpal tunnel syndrome, for example, is a disability. However, if the employer perceives it as a disability, it may be considered one.

In a recent case, the Equal Employment Opportunity Commission alleged that an employer violated the ADA by withdrawing a job offer to a punch-press operator after learning of the applicant's history of carpal tunnel syndrome. The employer claimed that the applicant wasn't disabled under the law. However, a federal court in Illinois found that the employer had withdrawn the job offer precisely because it did consider carpal tunnel syndrome a disability. As such, the court ruled, the applicant must be considered disabled, and was allowed to pursue a claim of damages.

If you have been ruled permanently disabled by the worker's compensation system, that does not mean you are automatically considered disabled under the law. However, it is relevant evidence.

What Constitutes Discrimination?

Various circumstances are specifically covered by the ADA. If an employer refuses to make a reasonable accommodation, that would likely be considered a cause for action. Remember, however, that the employer must know about the need for accommodation, so it is incumbent upon you to ask for it.

Limiting an employee's opportunities because of a disability is illegal. That means you cannot be denied a promotion or raise because of your disability. As with other cases of discrimination, this can be difficult to prove. In addition, an employer who enters into an agreement that might subject disabled employees to discrimination is violating the law.

Finally, the ADA bars an employer from denying equal job benefits to the disabled, which means you should not be forced to pay more for health benefits, for example. Nor should you be denied any company disability benefits that are provided to other employees. Under the law, all employees must be treated the same.

What Is Permissible
Before You Are Hired?

If you are applying for a job, an employer is not allowed to ask if you have a disability, or if you have ever received worker's compensation. However, the employer can ask if you are able to perform the essential functions of the job. No medical exam is permitted before you are offered a job.

Once a job offer is made, the company can require you to undergo a medical exam. Many, if not most, companies do this. However, all applicants must have the same exam. If an employer decides to withdraw a job offer based on the results of the medical exam, the employer must show that you are not capable of performing the essential functions of the job. Any information about your disability must be kept confidential, in separate medical files. Your supervisor, as well as safety personnel, may be informed, but only to facilitate any accommodations you may need.

If You Decide to Sue

An insurance-company executive, who is also a medical doctor, noticed the pains in his hands after he spent long hours typing evaluations of policyholders' claims. Eventually, his own doctors ordered him to leave work, and performed surgery on his hands. Despite the surgeries, his hands are still painful, weak, and spastic, limiting his ability to work and take care of himself. He has been diagnosed with reflex sympathetic dystrophy, and fears that he will be unable to find significant medical work anywhere else. Desperate, he decided to sue his former employer under the Americans With Disabilities Act.

Under the act, qualified disabled workers who believe they have been subjected to discrimination may file suit through the Equal Employment Opportunity Commission. The law stipulates that you cannot sue your employer under the ADA without the commission's approval. The commission is not required to accept every case. There is a cap on permitted damages, ranging from $50,000 to $300,000. You also have up to a hundred and eighty days after the alleged discrimination occurred in which to file a claim. Lawyers who specialize in disability issues emphasize the need for filing a claim while you are still on the job because it protects you from retaliation through termination or demotion.

If you win, you are entitled to a remedy that would place you in a job position that you would have held had there been no discrimination. You may also be entitled to back pay and attorney's fees.

If the commission declines your case, you may be able to sue under a variety of state laws. One microfilmer, who had to place papers under a camera lens and push a button to photograph them 14,500 times a day, won $1.2 million after a court in Washington state ruled that her employer had violated state disability law by not providing her with better work conditions after she developed tendinitis.

RSI does not automatically qualify as a disability under the ADA. Whether it is considered a disability depends on the facts of the particular situation. In addition, if RSI prevents you from doing the essential functions of your job, you may not have protection. In January 1990, the U.S. District Court in the southern district of Alabama ruled that the dismissal of a postal worker with carpal tunnel syndrome was proper because his injury prevented him from being able to do the essential functions of his job.

Legal action can take years before you see results. In addition, the outcome is impossible to predict. It could also brand you as a troublemaker. Filing suit is an extreme step; many people involved in legal actions say that it takes an emotional toll as well.

What the ADA Doesn't Do

The law does not protect you if you cannot perform the essential functions of the job, with or without accommodation. It does not guarantee you a job, or protect you from layoff. The law is designed to open doors and prevent discrimination, but you must prove you are qualified for the job. If several qualified applicants are competing for the same job, the employer is not compelled to give it to the disabled applicant.

Steps Employers Should Take to Comply with the ADA

There has been much publicity about how to comply with the law, and even a few scams, but there are some basic steps employers should take. They include the following:

- *Make sure interviewers are trained.* Because questions about a person's disability are specifically barred under the law, interviewers should be trained about what questions to avoid. They should also be told that they can ask about a person's ability to perform the essential functions of a job.
- *Eliminate illegal language on company forms.* All job applications and other company forms should be reviewed to eliminate illegal questions. Illegal questions include "Do you have any physical or mental disabilities that would affect your ability to perform the job?" or "Have you ever filed a worker's compensation claim?"
- *Do not make medical judgments.* Any employer concerned about a person's ability to do a job should rely on qualified medical advice.

- *Develop job descriptions.* Written job descriptions are one form of evidence of the essential functions of a job.
- *Review the company's employment physical exams.* Pre-employment physicals are not permitted under the law. They are only allowed after a job offer has been made.
- *Maintain confidentiality of records.* Procedures should be in place to prevent disclosure of medical records.
- *Be flexible.* As mentioned previously, most accommodations for the disabled require little or no cost.

Employers who hire disabled workers are entitled to certain benefits, including the Targeted Jobs Tax Credit, which is a credit against tax liability. Grants are also available to employers seeking to modify the workplace to better accommodate disabled workers.

In addition, several occupational studies have documented a significant drop in worker's compensation and other medical costs after companies institute ergonomic modifications. Most changes are easy and relatively inexpensive. Given the savings they often bring, they add up to good business.

❧
RETURN TO WORK

If you have been forced out of work because of your RSI, one of the best ways to protect your rights is to get back to work. This is not to say that you should return before you are physically ready, but employees on the job are always treated better than those on disability. If you are receiving worker's compensation, you are a liability to your company. If you are able to return to work, you considerably reduce the cost of your case to your employer.

If you are not physically capable of doing your old job, you may be able to handle an alternative job. Try to come up with possibilities that will make sense to your employer. It takes creativity and flexibility, but some companies have successfully provided alternative work to employees.

Returning to work not only helps protect your rights, but it's also good for your state of mind. Although some injured workers abhor the thought of returning to the place that injured them, others relish the opportunity to be productive again. Most employers would rather have an injured worker being productive on the job rather than at home not working.

TAKE CHARGE

Many people with RSI complain that dealing with the legal, employment, and insurance issues of their injury is like having a full-time job. Worse, it's like having a job where you constantly feel angry. It's hard to accept the fundamental unfairness of having to fight for benefits if you've been injured on the job. The systems designed to protect workers are complicated and confusing, but, ultimately, they provide essential protections to workers. To take advantage of them and to protect your rights, you must be informed and take an active role in making sure you get what you are due. Just as you must take an active role in your recovery, you must be in charge of protecting yourself. It's a lot of work, but you will be better off, both financially and emotionally.

CHAPTER 14

OPENING
NEW DOORS

❧

Liz remembers pain so "excruciating" that she couldn't work at her job as a copy editor. Initially misdiagnosed with carpal tunnel syndrome, she later was correctly diagnosed—after many tests and visits to other doctors—with myofascial pain syndrome. It was serious enough for her doctor to tell her to stop typing altogether.

Being unable to type meant that she couldn't work because her job consisted of intensive computer keyboard work. Her Minneapolis employer was supportive and came up with a "make-work" job that allowed her to continue to work. Like many people with RSI, Liz couldn't bear the thought of being unemployed. "I was so anxious. I couldn't imagine what I'd do if I couldn't come to work," she says.

She was also angry, she says, "at a corporate culture that could allow this to happen to good workers." After nine months of trying a range of treatments, from physical therapy and biofeedback to swimming, Liz was able to resume limited typing and do editing work that required less time at the computer keyboard. She also became active in her union, the Newspaper Guild, pushing hard to make her company aware of the need for training programs and ergonomic equipment.

That time, in the early 1990s, was painful and difficult for Liz. "Your faith is shaken in so many things you believe in," she says. But it also forced her to look at some issues in her personal life and to make some changes. Once she was healthy enough, she and her husband took a three-month leave from work and traveled through Europe, an experience that profoundly changed her perspective on life. She has since changed career directions and now works for the Newspaper Guild in Silver Spring, Maryland, as editor of the union's monthly paper, The Guild Reporter.

Liz is proud of the changes she helped push through at her former job, and she's happy to be doing work that allows her to be an advocate for other workers. She is also convinced that her experience with RSI helped her reach this point. "I'm sure I wouldn't be doing this and be the person that I am if it wasn't for that struggle," she says.

❈
CHANGE IS INEVITABLE

The very nature of RSI forces you to change. Whether it's a simple matter of changing how you work or it is something more, like changing jobs, you probably will have to confront change. Many of the people interviewed for this book talked about the positive changes they were forced to make as a result of RSI; everyone who did so said they were happy they had to change. This chapter will discuss some of the changes individuals made and the steps you can take if you choose to change your job or career.

Change is unsettling. It's not easy, and it often involves risk. You exchange a comfortable, familiar existence for something new and uncertain. Although it may be a cliché, there is truth in the statement that for every door that closes, another opens. It may be hard to see that if you are in the throes of dealing with your injury and fighting an unsympathetic employer or worker's compensation system. The fact is, though, that with RSI, you really have no choice but to deal with change, so take an active rather than passive role.

❃
CHANGING JOBS

Over and over, people with RSI who were interviewed for this book talked about changing jobs. Some did it simply because they could no longer handle the physical demands of their former positions. Others did it because they couldn't bear the thought of returning to work for an employer they felt had injured them. Still others simply had no choice—they were fired or laid off because of their injury. And others discovered interests that were more satisfying, and chose to pursue them.

If you are considering changing jobs, basically two avenues are open to you: You can switch to a related job; or you can change careers altogether. Either choice involves enormous upheaval, but it is not uncommon in today's changing marketplace. You'll find you have a lot of company on this road.

Changing to a Related Job

It is easy to develop tunnel vision about job options when you are busy juggling work and personal responsibilities. If you are considering a job change, you obviously need to spend time thinking about and researching other jobs. Job counselors talk about "job clusters," that is, occupations that are related to one another. For example, a media job cluster would include everything from electronic technician and reporter to producer. Or a marketing job cluster might include everything from sales agent and package designer to direct-mail agent.

If you are hoping to change to a job that uses skills you already have but which will not place the physical demands on you that your current job does, look around your company to see if there are openings that might be a fit for you. If you are worried about discussing this with your supervisor, you might seek out a supervisor you trust in another department or area and ask for confidential advice.

It may be a matter of leaving your company and marketing the skills you have differently. Andy, the Ann Arbor, Michigan-based Webmaster, developed RSI after working long hours in a highly pressured environment at a computer company. He typed "around the clock" on the job, creating a new Website every day. A fast typist—he types ninety to a hundred words a minute—the pains and spasms he suddenly felt in his hands and forearms brought him up short. "When you first get it, it's just terrifying, especially if you're a guy, because your identity is so entwined with doing your job," he says.

Andy decided to start his own company with a partner and has found it to be far more satisfying and profitable as well. He has created his own Web page on RSI (http://webreference.com/rsi.html). It starts off like this:

So there I was at my Mac, typing away at the Great American Novel.

> *"I was nursing my third bourbon, my contact was late, and my wisdom tooth was acting up again. A hush fell over the bar as a stunning blond appeared. Every eye in the place followed her. She swayed her hips suggestively as she sidled up to me at the bar. As casually as I could, I glanced her way. I clinked the ice in my glass—twice. I knew my contact's name was Alex, but I didn't realize 'he' was a 'she'.* This changes everything, *I thought."*

> *Suddenly a sharp, searing pain shot up my right arm. I completely forgot about Alex and her troubles and concentrated on mine.*
> *I clutched my arm, massaged it a bit, and kept on typing (mistake). I ended up in the emergency room and found that I probably had an RSI (Repetitive Strain Injury). The doctor prescribed ice packs, rest, and a double dose of Aleve.*

The page continues with his story and advice to others on RSI. Andy created the RSI Web page, he says, because, "I thought I could help other people."

He now has his symptoms under control but admits to a "lingering concern" about RSI. But he is happy with the change he made because of it. "It forces you to slow down," he says. "You have no choice."

Following are some other examples of people with RSI who have made changes to related jobs:

- A secretary who was seriously debilitated by carpal tunnel syndrome now sets up computers for her employer. She admits that it's "ironic," but loves doing it because she's good at it. Although it is a completely new set of skills, she's still working for the same employer.
- A journalist laid off from his job because of his tendinitis switched to a public relations job in which he spends far less time on a computer keyboard and far more time in strategic-planning sessions. He finds it more interesting and much more lucrative.
- A medical-claims processor no longer able to do her job because of an array of RSIs now teaches classes to aspiring municipal employees who are studying for Civil Service exams. She finds working with people far more satisfying, but admits she doesn't make as much money.

Making such changes requires some thought and work. Talk to a career counselor or vocational rehabilitation specialist. Many states provide free counseling services to the disabled.

Changing Careers

Changing careers may seem like a more ambitious endeavor, but job marketing specialists say that most people will change careers at least two to three times in a lifetime of working. Sometimes it takes working in one or two transitional jobs before you move into one that is right for you. Sometimes it requires additional education or training to acquire the skills you need. It almost always takes a little research and perseverance, but those who've done it say the rewards are well worth it.

John was a thirty-two-year-old computer programmer when he was injured for a second time. His company was supportive and hired transcribers so that he could dictate computer programs without having to type. Though grateful for the help, he found dictating to another person frustrating and painstakingly difficult. "It just took all the fun out of it," he says. After about a year, he left the company and focused on his own business of publishing a directory of translation agencies. He doesn't type; instead, he uses voice-recognition software. Although John says he probably would have left computer programming anyway, RSI spurred him to work full time on his own business, which he enjoys. He likes getting the chance to do his own advertising, bookkeeping, and contracts and adds, "It just matters to you so much more when it's your own business."

Following are some examples of RSI sufferers who chose to make drastic career changes as a result of their injuries:

- A lawyer who developed sharp pains in his wrists and shoulders after long hours at his computer started his own company marketing ergonomic equipment. The company has yet to make money, but he feels he's doing something positive.
- A writer who felt she could no longer spend many hours at a computer keyboard got a degree in social work. She now counsels people with a wide range of problems and believes her experiences help her bring a special dimension to therapy. She says she has never been happier.
- A postal worker who believes she was forced to quit her job because of her RSI has started a direct-mail business with her family. She says it's fun and makes money.

All of these people had to do some planning before they made those changes. If you want to make a similar change, many books can provide a wealth of practical information on how to go about it. Check your local library. There are also companies that will—for a fee—create a résumé, develop interviewing skills, and even help you decide what you want to do. You may be able to get the same advice for free from your local vocational rehabilitation department. Sometimes, colleges and universities have career counselors who offer free counseling and other assistance to the disabled.

Steps to Take When Changing Jobs

Once you get started, there are some basic steps you should take. They include looking at your experience, taking time to dream, assessing your skills and interests, narrowing and researching your choices, and thinking about the physical demands of any job in which you might be interested. It can be a fascinating experience that can lead you to an exciting opportunity.

Look at your experience Don't view your experience solely in terms of job skills. Think about the things you've done that you've found to be particularly satisfying. There may be a personal or volunteer experience that was particularly meaningful. Write them down. Analyze why you found those experiences satisfying. Once you do that, you'll have important clues as to the kind of work you would most enjoy doing.

Dream Don't be afraid to explore something you've always fantasized about doing but never could for one reason or another. This is the time to think about those fantasies and see if you can make one a reality. Bear in mind, though, that as you explore it further, your "dream job" may not be what you think it is. You may find that a second or third career choice is much better suited to your interests and needs.

Realistically assess your skills and interests   You may do this through a career-counseling test or an exercise in one of the many books available on the subject. Don't write this off, assuming that you already know what you're interested in doing and what you are able to do. If you take the time to explore this, through a test or a written exercise or in a session with a counselor, you may discover some possibilities you had never considered.

Narrow your career or job choices, and research them   Go to the library and read about the occupations in which you are interested. Check out the occupational forecasts put out by the federal government. It's fine to decide that a particular occupation is right for you, but if there are few or no jobs available, you may be setting yourself up for frustration and rejection. Two particularly good sources of information on this are the *Dictionary of Occupational Titles* (Washington, D.C.: U.S. Department of Labor, Employment and Training Administration, U.S. Employment Service) and the *Occupational Outlook Handbook* (Washington, D.C.: U.S. Department of Labor, Bureau of Labor Statistics). They are likely to be available in the reference section of your library.

You also want to find out if a particular company is sensitive to ergonomic issues and RSI. One large computer company actually has a room filled with ergonomic equipment and an array of keyboards for employees to try out. Others concerned about the spread of RSI have made modifications to try to prevent it. A company like that might be a good fit for you.

Once you narrow your choices to a certain company or companies, you can read the annual reports—they're often available in college or business libraries. An even easier source of information is your daily newspaper or local business journal. If the company is at all prominent, there will be a host of stories about it. To read back issues, simply go to your local library. Many newspapers have on-line services available to the public as well.

Think about the physical demands of the job   Unless you are familiar with the new occupation in which you are seeking a job, you may be surprised by what it requires physically. One newspaper journalist was persuaded by a career counselor to go into television reporting to take advantage of the skills she already had and to cut down on the time she spent typing. The woman dutifully took television-reporting classes and contacted local television stations. She was finally offered a reporting job, but it required that she do her own camera and sound work. Because of her RSI, it was physically impossible for her to carry a television camera and sound equipment all day long. She had to abandon the idea.

To assess these physical demands adequately, you may need to see an occupational therapist, who can advise you and also help you work out ways you can physically accomplish a job. Bear in mind that you will get better with time and that activities you cannot manage now will probably be manageable later. Don't give up!

GETTING A JOB

Getting a new job takes work. Do what any job-seeker would do: Read recruitment ads in your local newspaper or professional publications, contact job-placement services when appropriate, write letters, and network like crazy. Many excellent books detail how to get a job; consult them for more specifics on these skills. Check your local library or bookstore.

Rather than discuss those skills here, it's more important to discuss the big issue that faces anyone with RSI who is seeking a new job: Should you disclose your condition to a prospective employer?

Disclosing Your RSI

This is tricky. Many advocates for the disabled—and RSI is often included in that category—argue strongly that if you disclose your injury, you won't get the job. However, if you don't disclose, that sets up a different set of problems. Consider the case of the woman who did not tell the company that hired her that she had RSI until after she started work. It came up only after she requested some special ergonomic equipment and explained that she needed it for her arms and hands. Her employer provided the equipment and she set about doing her job—and doing it well, she thought. In time, however, she began to hear some backbiting comments about her not disclosing her condition, that she had somehow been deceitful. Although she did not hear direct complaints about her work, her relationship with the man who hired her became increasingly strained. Eventually, she was laid off. Today, she is convinced that her decision not to disclose her physical limitations poisoned the well for her at that job.

But, as many people with disabilities know, she was in a bind. Prejudice against people with disabilities runs high. Employers worry about whether disabled people can do the job. They worry about liability. They worry that disabled workers will be less reliable or will require expensive accommodations. They worry about increased insurance rates. All of these are prejudices that are rarely spoken, but they may be considerations. If you disclose your injury, you may be ruled out of a job without ever getting the chance to address any of these issues.

That means you have a choice: You can take your chances and not disclose your injury. If you don't require special accommodations but merely request an ergonomic workstation, you may be able to pull it off without incident. If you require more than that, you risk leaving your employer with the feeling that you were dishonest when you interviewed for the job. Any working relationship is built on a number of things, not the least of which is trust. If you don't disclose your disability, you will have a tough time establishing that trust.

If you decide to disclose it, there are any number of opportunities along the way when you can do it fairly gracefully. You can, for example, put it on your résumé, if there's a positive association with it, such as running a peer support group for people with RSI. It may also be a way to cover a gap in your résumé if your condition temporarily forced you out of work. One résumé tip: Most job-seekers now specify only the specific years they were employed at a particular job, not the months, which is a way to cover a brief period of unemployment.

Additionally, if you think any experience you've had because of your injury will be a plus for the job for which you are applying, you could mention it in a cover letter. One woman became so concerned about educating others about RSI that she set up a national clearinghouse for information on it. She met professionals from across the country and gained invaluable experience in organizing a conference on it. That kind of experience could be a plus worth mentioning, both in a résumé and cover letter.

The question might arise on a job application. Even though it is illegal to ask you about a disability on a job application, some forms still have questions like, "Do you have any physical limitations that would hinder you in any way from performing the job?" That is probably an illegal question, but it does you no good to point that out. If you can perform the job with reasonable accommodations, you can honestly answer that question with "No."

A prospective employer can ask you in a job interview whether you have any physical limitations that prevent you from performing essential functions of the job. As with the job application, if you can work with reasonable accommodations, you can truthfully answer "No," but you probably will want to ask whether the company supplies ergonomic equipment to employees. (Many companies do.)

This is an opportunity to raise the issue of your RSI. Try to frame it in as positive a way as possible. Try to talk about it casually. Talking about ergonomic equipment might be a natural way to do it. Often, people who have never had symptoms of RSI have seen other people who have and are sufficiently worried about it and want to know how to protect themselves. They could be eager to hear any information you have about preventing it. One man, who was nervous about bringing up his injury—which was mostly under control—was stunned when he mentioned a piece of ergonomic equipment he preferred, that his interviewer immediately wrote down the particulars because she had just begun experiencing symptoms herself! (He was offered the job, but turned it down in favor of a better one.) Remember, RSI is an equal-opportunity injury. It strikes everyone, from lower-level employees to managers.

Some advocates for the disabled say the best time to disclose a disability is after a job offer has been made but *before* you've accepted it. They argue that you have a better chance of getting the job if you hold off disclosing the disability until the job offer is made. It also makes it more difficult—probably illegal—for the employer to withdraw the offer after learning of your disability. If you do this, talk about it matter-of-factly and make a point of saying that it will have no effect on your ability to do a good job; then restate the skills that got you the job offer in the first place. One point, however: This timing can backfire. The employer may feel *had*. You have to judge whether it's the right timing.

Whether or not to disclose your injury is a highly personal decision. Think about it before going to your interview, and rehearse what you might say. You must get a feel for the interviewer to determine whether this is the right place and time to talk about it.

Getting a copy of the job description for your desired position can be a helpful guide on how to pitch your skills and experience to a prospective employer, as well as discern the essential functions of the job. You could try to get one by calling the company's human resources department, but many departments consider job descriptions internal documents and won't give them out. Sometimes job descriptions are posted in public employment offices and community centers.

If you decide to disclose your RSI, try to address any concerns you think the employer might have. For example, if you think a prospective employer is worried that if you are hired, the company's insurance rates will go up—probably the number one concern—you can explain that health, life, and worker's compensation insurance companies do not raise premiums just because someone with a disability is added to a group policy. Many factors are considered when setting premium rates. In addition, if the company is a large one, any increase that might occur would be spread over a big enough pool of employees so that premiums would not be affected.

Again, all of this is tricky. Whether you get the job may depend more on your passion and enthusiasm.

✄

POLITICAL CHANGE

Advocates for people with RSI say they've seen a real change in the political landscape in recent years. More and more people are familiar with it, the medical community has made strides in educating its members about it, and many employers are making ergonomic changes in the workplace. "The RSI epidemic really was just a matter of time, as jobs have become so computer-intensive," says Hilary Marcus, of the Coalition on New Office Technology in Boston. The CNOT, started in 1987 by office workers concerned about the effects of office technology on health and worker rights, advocates for injured and at-risk workers. It gets calls from all over the country about RSI, Marcus says.

That change has touched the political landscape as well. In the early 1990s, it was a fairly obscure issue, but since then, it's become "basically a political hot potato," says Michael Gauf, managing editor of *CTD News*, a monthly newsletter on the latest developments affecting RSI. He attributes that change to the increase in knowledge and reporting of RSI. "RSI is more recognizable now."

Many states and local municipalities have proposed legislation that would compel employers to provide ergonomic equipment and rest breaks to VDT users. Although several such laws have passed, only to be vetoed or overturned by the courts, the sentiment is still strong that regulations are needed to protect workers. In fact, in 1997 the state of California passed a law that would require any employer to implement an ergonomics program if more than one employee reports identical RSIs—diagnosed by a physician—in identical work. The law broadly defines an ergonomics program to include looking for risk factors, changing job design, correcting ergonomic problems, and training employees. Other states are closely watching the California law to see if it is upheld.

On the federal level, the U.S. Occupational Safety and Health Administration has resumed plans to push for a federal ergonomics standard. When the federal government first released a draft standard in the early 1990s, it ran into stiff opposition mounted by a well-organized coalition of businesses. They lobbied hard against the regulation, arguing that it would be unwise and costly, without helping injured workers. Budget legislation prohibiting such a standard stalled OSHA until 1997, when officials announced plans to resume developing a standard. There is still some opposition in Congress to such a standard, but OSHA has created a new position, ergonomics coordinator, to oversee educational activities, research, enforcement, and rule-making.

That move, say some observers, is important because it keeps the issue at the forefront. The first time a standard was released, a whole new wave of businesses specializing in ergonomic and other RSI-related products opened up, Gauf says. Some of those companies closed or cut back their product lines after the standard appeared to have been defeated, but he expects a resurgence of entrepreneurial interest now that the push is on again for a federal standard.

Unions see businesses banding together again to fight any ergonomics standard. This fight is tougher, and more ferocious than other workplace health and safety battles because managers see an ergonomics rule as encroaching on their right to manage, says Nancy Lessin, senior staff for strategy and policy at Mass COSH, the Massachusetts Coalition for Occupational Safety and Health, one of twenty-four nonprofit committees across the country working on behalf of worker safety and health. It's not just a matter of buying proper equipment, Lessin says, it's also one of job design—a touchy area for managers who believe they have the right to determine staffing levels, work pace and production quotas. Lessin says management's rights to manage never includes the right to injure workers.

Even without a federal ergonomics standard, OSHA has been actively involved in preventing RSI in the workplace. It has sued more than four hundred companies for having dangerous conditions that led to RSIs. OSHA investigates workplace conditions in response to signed, written complaints. However, any response to a complaint about RSI is likely to take time because the agency investigates workplaces in order of priority, with life-threatening conditions ranking first.

If you feel there are dangerous conditions in your workplace and your employer has not responded to worker complaints, you can write to your regional OSHA office. Any letter should include your company's name and address, the nature of the problem in as much detail as possible, how long the problem has existed, and your name and a place where an OSHA representative can contact you. If you want your complaint to be formally considered, you must sign the letter. If you do not, OSHA will not consider it a formal complaint and will merely send a letter to the company that it has been notified of a problem. OSHA is required by law not to reveal your name. Contact the main office by writing to the Occupational Safety and Health Administration, 1825 K Street, NW, Washington, DC 20006. (More details on OSHA listed in the appendix.)

Government interest has been sparked by the continuing rise in the number of cases and by union involvement as well. Both the AFL-CIO and the Communication Workers of America have come out strongly in trying to protect workers with RSI. They've lobbied for protective legislation, worked to get language in union contracts, and even been involved in some important research on the subject.

RSI also has become one of the more higher-profile issues addressed by the Committees on Occupational Safety and Health. These are nonprofit organizations, located throughout the United States, whose staffers work to help protect workers' health. They work closely with labor unions and spend time lobbying on behalf of workers. Staff members can provide you with information, names of doctors, and names of lawyers specializing in workplace law. (For a list of all the COSH groups, see the appendix.)

The Coalition on New Office Technology has an RSI ACTION campaign that emphasizes education, outreach, and advocacy. Working with other local and national groups, it has organized petition drives and rallies. Despite the increasing awareness of RSI, it is still difficult for injured workers to get information, CNOT's Marcus says.

Many of these advocacy groups are eager for volunteers and draw on people with RSI for help. "When injured workers are hurt and they need support," Marcus says, "this is a great way to do something positive with anger." She adds, however, that many of their volunteers are available only temporarily and then move on with their lives.

There is nothing wrong with that. Take from the experience any positives you can. Dealing with RSI can be maddening, frustrating, and tedious, but it also can offer new opportunities.

A PERSONAL STORY

❖

SANDRA'S STORY

I am writing this book on an alternative keyboard, one that breaks into three parts and angles upward. It's the only keyboard I can use without feeling an immediate, burning pain in my arms. Even with this ergonomically designed keyboard, a custom-made wrist rest, and other ergonomic adaptations, my neck hurts and my forearms are starting to ache. I'll have to take a break soon and return to dictating later. The pains don't worry me much; I've had far, far worse with RSI. At one point in my life, not so long ago, I was so crippled by this nasty injury that I could not drive my car, write a check, or lift a teacup.

Though it now seems like a lifetime ago, and I guess it was, I remember vividly when I first felt it—the afternoon of October 6, 1989. There was no warning, nothing to prepare me for the intensity or suddenness of the pain. I've since had two children, and the pain of RSI was worse than labor.

It all began with a flame of pain searing my left arm. Startled, I pulled my hands away from my computer keyboard, where I had been editing a Sunday story. As assistant editor for *Newsday*, the paper of record for Long Island, New York, such chores were routine. I had logged many hours on that keyboard, and Friday afternoons were particularly long because of the extra copy. I shook my arm and tried to resume typing, but it was like putting my hands on a branding iron. I had to stop.

Like many of my friends with RSI, I am dedicated to my work. I love it. Like my colleagues, I had worked hard to land my job. At the time, nothing could have stopped me from doing it—except, of course, a pain so intense I couldn't continue.

I scanned our vast newsroom, thinking it would somehow help me understand what had just happened. But that day, I saw nothing unusual. Phones rang, computer terminals clicked, and staffers talked about stories for the next day's paper. It was an ordinary day, yet something extraordinary had just happened to me.

My boss was surprised when I told him I would finish my work the next day. So was I. I never left early. But on this particular Friday I had no choice. I went home, but my arms continued to burn through the night, the next day, and the next night and day. By Tuesday, I was in the white-walled examining room of a doctor's office. He calmly diagnosed tendinitis in both arms and carpal tunnel syndrome. Because he didn't seem worried, I wasn't; but I still was in constant pain.

"What do I do about the pain?" I asked.

He advised me to cut back on my typing, but he couldn't tell me by how much or how I was supposed to complete my work without typing. He couldn't give me many answers. It frustrated me, but I would soon learn that frustration would be my constant companion. Few people would be able to give me specific answers. I would have to find them myself.

I left the doctor's office with a prescription for ibuprofen, 1,800 milligrams a day, to ease the pain. As I gripped the steering wheel I felt my fingers go numb. I dismissed it. I had just seen a doctor. I would do what he told me to do, and everything would be OK.

I was wrong, of course. Even though I cut back on my typing at work, the pain was constant. A few weeks later, I dropped my hairbrush. I had to scoop it up with both hands and found I couldn't grip it. I couldn't hold a toothbrush or fold a paper bag. This time, I panicked. I called the doctor, who advised me to stay out of work for three weeks and prescribed 2,400 milligrams a day of ibuprofen.

Pain surged through my body like an electric current. Every movement I made seemed to inflame my arms. I tried to calm them down by sitting still. I couldn't read because turning pages hurt too much, so I watched television and walked. But nothing seemed to help. Even the ibuprofen only took the edge off the pain. I felt trapped.

Merlin, my boisterous Labrador retriever, immediately sensed a problem. He refused to let me out of his sight. He had never been a particularly serious watchdog—he had never been particularly serious about anything—but now he was vigilant, barking at anything that moved past our house. Whenever I answered the door, instead of bolting outside, he would sit quietly next to me.

I decided to tackle my problem by changing what I could: diet and exercise. Although I had always been careful about both, I consulted a nutritionist and resumed running every day. Merlin was my running companion and he was delighted with our new routine. The exercise was a tonic for me, too. It was the only time of day I wasn't aware of my arms burning.

When I returned to work, I tentatively typed a few words on the computer. After a total of no more than twenty keystrokes, my arms burned again. The burning continued until 2 A.M. the next day. I tried to keep working and again called my doctor, who was sympathetic but unable to offer answers. He prescribed another painkiller.

I was desperately trying to fulfill my responsibilities on the job and at home, but I could barely make it through the day. Several colleagues, seeing what I was going through, urged me to see another doctor. I did, Dr. Craig Rosenberg, who has tended my arms since then and shepherded this book to completion. In our first meeting, he was calm, kind, and thorough. Though I stupidly tried to downplay my pain, I could see by the look in his eyes that he got it. He knew it was real and that I was in trouble. He immediately prescribed splints to immobilize my arms temporarily, as well as occupational therapy. He explained that while typing had caused my injury, I had to rest my arms as much as possible. I needed to stop driving, and cut back on housework, and cut back on any use of my arms. And he acknowledged that my case was not a mild one.

His advice confirmed what I already knew. I had already stopped driving because my arms burned so much I couldn't grip the wheel. And although I had never been an avid housekeeper, now even the basics were too daunting. But Rosenberg had given me something important: hope and direction. He gave me something to do to effect my recovery. Waiting passively for the pain simply to fade was driving me crazy because it never did. Now, at least, I had a direction, and the hope that I could deal with the problem.

I found an occupational therapist who asked me to take a test that included adjectives to describe my pain. I found myself circling words like *searing* and *burning*. By the time I was finished, both she and I were stunned. I had never used those words in talking to her about my pain. I had minimized it. To my mind, complaining was unseemly. I grew up in Minnesota, where the long, harsh winters and Scandinavian temperament encourage self-sufficiency and stoicism. I had always prided myself on those qualities and felt deeply uncomfortable asking for help. I learned later that many of my compatriots in this injury are exactly the same way.

My therapist set about making me splints, massaging my arms, and teaching me how to do contrast baths at home. I did them religiously, four times a day, and they did relieve the pain. I would immerse my arms four minutes in warm water, and then one minute in ice-cold water four times for a total of twenty minutes. I started feeling better, but still found that seemingly mundane tasks would start the pain again. Pushing buttons on the phone, which I used throughout the workday, became impossible. So my therapist devised a solution. She stuck a pencil through a foam rubber ball for me, and I pressed the buttons with the eraser end of the pencil. It worked beautifully, but my coworkers were shocked at how weak I had become.

For a while, I thought I could pull the whole thing off. I thought I could work at a demanding job and deal with an injury that was just as demanding. But despite putting all my energy into both, my condition worsened. I simply couldn't juggle both; I wasn't getting enough rest for my arms. By May 1990, I was unable to feed or dress myself. If someone had told me a year earlier that this would happen to me—me, the intrepid, self-sufficient journalist—I would have laughed and said that was impossible. But it wasn't, and I was living it.

I had to leave work and go on disability, beginning a years-long odyssey to restore my health. It involved trying a range of therapies, from traditional to alternative, exercising, and coping with the anger, frustration, and humiliation of becoming a second-class citizen. Because like it or not, that's what I was while on disability: a second-class citizen. I was lucky; most of my friends and coworkers were sympathetic. My employer believed me because many other people at the paper had been similarly afflicted. But when you are dealing with worker's compensation and other systems like it, you are treated a bit differently. Some doctors don't want to deal with you, and even the most well-intentioned of friends couldn't help telling me that I must have done something to cause my injury.

RSI brought out in me an extraordinary intensity of emotion. I remember days of raging at insurance-company functionaries when my bills weren't paid. That rage wasn't me; I normally am an easygoing person. But the fundamental unfairness of my being so badly injured by my work was hard to swallow. I had been brought up to believe that if I worked hard, I would get ahead. Instead, I was crippled.

Then there were the nightmares. I had forgotten about them until a friend with RSI recently mentioned that she'd dreamt of her hand being caught in a garbage disposal. During my worst period of pain and disability, I would wake up screaming at least once a week. It was always the same dream: A man was trying to cut off my arms with a machete. Every time, I would wake up screaming, "No, no, no!"

Of all the things I experienced because of my RSI—the pain, loss of functioning, isolation, loss of income, professional status, and even the loss of some friends—more than anything I hated being treated as if I were somehow inferior. People I didn't know well felt they could ask me the most intimate questions about my personal health and state of mind. Some doctors felt they could take on a smug, condescending tone. And some insurance-company representatives felt they could simply dismiss me.

One day, in a huff over something like that, I was talking with my worker's compensation lawyer, a smart, funny guy who is genuinely interested in workers' rights. I am embarrassed to tell this story because it reflects badly on me, but it makes an important point. I told my lawyer that I wasn't some malingerer trying to fake an injury to get out of work. I wasn't a construction worker. I was a professional dedicated to my work, my calling, and I should not be treated as anything less. His eyes narrowed just a bit, and he said quietly, "Ninety-nine percent of the people who file worker's compensation claims have real injuries and want to work. They're not faking."

It brought me up short. Ashamed, I realized there are no class divisions with RSI. I wouldn't have cared about them even if there were. I had fallen victim to the same kind of prejudices that so deeply offended me when directed at me. I resolved never to make that mistake again.

I learned other lessons from my RSI. Most of them weren't terribly dramatic; I can't say that I've acquired any startling revelations about the meaning of life or changed my basic values in any way. If anything, the experience has brought me back to my core values. But I do see life a little differently. I think I see things that other people who haven't had this experience tend to miss. I can see both pain and courage in a person's eyes. I find nobility and grace in unexpected places. My life is richer; more textured. I hope I extend to others the compassion that has been extended to me.

Thank God I had a caring doctor and caring therapists. My massage therapist, Karen DeSimone, was single-minded about getting me back to health. Her selfless efforts on my behalf helped sustain me in more ways than she'll ever know. As someone who suffered from the pain of fibromyalgia herself, she understood what I was going through. She had the uncanny ability to touch my arms and immediately know what kind of pain I was in. I never even had to tell her. When I think of her, my doctor, and the other people who helped me get better, I am in awe of their caring and devotion. Healing is an art.

Chronic pain and disability change your life. Though the attitudes of others may not change, mine has. Certain friendships have been cemented by this experience; others have faded. I have learned about the kindness of strangers and the unintended cruelty of colleagues. My love and admiration for my husband, who stayed with me throughout my ordeal, has deepened. He has had to shoulder more of a burden around the house, and he often resented it; but other times, he would see me struggling with something, and he would quietly walk over and do it for me. Sometimes, he'd feel enraged that this injury had invaded our lives and cost us so much emotionally and financially. But it never crossed his mind to leave.

I have returned to work after more than two years on disability and several false starts in trying to return. I now work in a different job, thanks to a sympathetic employer and a supervisor who was willing to take a chance on me. He told me he wanted my brains, not my arms. I was dubious, but decided to give it a try, and I feel back on track. My colleagues have been unfailingly supportive, careful to not let me overdo in my enthusiasm for the job. I still have limitations. I still must exercise and do therapy regularly. And there are still interests and hobbies I cannot consider pursuing because of the strain they would put on my hands and arms. But I have a normal life again, something in my worst moments I wasn't sure I would ever have again.

I never thought I'd write this book. It seemed too great a physical undertaking, and I really wasn't sure I wanted to think all of these issues again. A dear friend and colleague, Ginger Rothe, who also has been crippled by RSI, convinced me that writing a book like this would help others. I wasn't sure, but I know that writing it has helped. Even after all my years in physical therapy, I picked up a few tips on how to manage my own symptoms. And interviewing the people for this book has brought back a lot of my own memories—some painful, some touching. Though I never want to return to those dark days when I was so crippled that I couldn't fasten a button or open a door, I do want to carry with me the good things I've gained. And I want my children to understand that everyone deserves compassion. I realized again how frightening RSI can be, especially if you don't know where to turn. My hope is that my friend Ginger is right, that this book will help provide needed information and perhaps, a little hope, to others who need it.

It does get better.

SANDRA'S HUSBAND'S STORY

It's 10 P.M. My wife has just gotten off the phone with a friend with whom she had been discussing some aspect of RSI for the past forty-five minutes. The phone rings again almost immediately. It's another call about RSI. It seems that every time the phone rings, it has something to do with RSI. A friend who tried to call me once joked that he couldn't get through because the "1-800-RSI-hotline" was busy for two hours.

I am angry. I am tired of dealing with this. It's become the center of my wife's life—and mine, too. Yet, I feel guilty. My wife—in pain every day for the last several years—has demonstrated incredible courage in dealing with an injury that has made it at times difficult for her to even brush her hair. And it has irreparably damaged her promising career in journalism. I am peeved about a phone call. I tell myself I should not be so selfish. After all, she is the one who was crippled.

I am supposed to feel sympathy, compassion, and understanding. But it's sometimes hard to muster those feelings. And I don't hide my annoyance very well. When we have tried to discuss her condition, I am not infrequently told in an angry tone of voice that I "don't understand" what she is going through. That's certainly true on some level. I have never had RSI. But for a therapist, a guy who makes his living understanding others, that can be pretty hard to hear.

It's also hard to be on the receiving end of some of the

rage she feels about her condition. At times, I have deserved it. But at other times, I have felt as if I am just getting what was meant for someone else—sort of like the dog that gets kicked when the owner gets home from a rough day.

But my wife is normally not irritable. She has a sunny disposition by nature. Sometimes, she doesn't let on how much she is hurting. (Or is it that I just haven't been able to listen carefully enough?) Besides, the anger is just a screen for all the hurt and fear. When we have been able to put aside our anger, her pain and tears have touched me. We have grown closer in the last few years.

Often, I just block out how much this has affected us. And at other times, I think the injury was a blessing in disguise. At least her life isn't consumed by the newspaper anymore. There's now more balance in her life, and in our lives. It seems to have helped Sandra slow down a bit. We probably wouldn't have had children if she had kept going with her career.

But the anger always comes back. Her injury, her pain— it's all so unnecessary. In fifty years, people will be amazed that machines were built that injured those who worked on them. This has been the 1990s equivalent of people who got sick from installing asbestos insulation for a living.

Sometimes, it seems the worst of it is behind us. My wife is getting better. Maybe she'll be able to turn adversity to advantage by writing this book. Maybe we can just go on with our lives.

But then the phone rings.

RESOURCES

CATALOGS FOR ADAPTIVE AIDS

Able Ware
1-800-443-4926
Adaptive and rehabilitative aids.

Adapt Ability
1-800-288-9941
Adaptive aids aimed at older people.

AliMed
1-800-225-2610
One catalog has ergonomic and occupational health products.
Another has aids for daily living.

Flag House Rehabilitation
1-800-793-7900
Clinical, physical therapy, occupational therapy equipment,
and supplies.

Independence House
1-800-932-2120
Has a range of adaptive products for the home and work, from ergonomic cooking utensils to an angled board for reading materials.

North Coast Medical
1-800-821-9319
One catalog has ergonomics products, from chairs to tool grips, for the workplace. Another catalog has aids for activities of daily living, including cooking and personal care.

Sammons Preston and Enrichments
1-800-323-5547
Features a wide array of adaptive and rehabilitative aids, from book holders to jar openers.

Saunders ErgoSource
1-800-969-4374
Features ergonomic equipment for work, from adjustable-height tables to document holders.

Self Care
1-800-345-4021
Fitness and health products, including relaxation aids and home ergonomics products.

Smith & Nephew Rehabilitation
1-800-558-8633
Adaptive and rehabilitative aids.

❊
ALTERNATIVE THERAPIES

Acupuncture

American Academy of Medical Acupuncture
1-800-521-2262
Has a referral service with names of physicians who are also acupuncturists. To get a list, leave your name and address, and the group will send one.

National Acupuncture and Oriental Medicine Alliance
P.O. Box 77511
Seattle, WA 98177-0531
(206) 851-6896

National Commission for the Certification of Acupuncturists
P. O. Box 97075
Washington, DC 20090-7075
(202) 232-1404

Alexander Technique

**North American Society of Teachers
of the Alexander Technique**
3010 Hennepin Ave. S.
Minneapolis, MN 55408
1-800-473-0620
Has a list of certified teachers of the Alexander Technique, as well as books and information on the technique.

Biofeedback

Biofeedback Certification Institute of America
10200 West 44th Ave., Apt. 304
Wheat Ridge, CO 80033-8436
(303) 420-2902
Publishes a register of biofeedback practitioners. The entire register is available for a fee, but the institute will send you a free list of biofeedback practitioners in your area.

Chiropractic

American Chiropractic Association
1701 Clarendon Blvd.
Arlington, VA 22209
(703) 276-8800
Will provide you a list of chiropractors in your area.

Feldenkrais

Feldenkrais Guild
P.O. Box 489
Albany, OR 97321-0143
1-800-775-2118
E-mail: feldngld@peak.org
Website: http:\\www.feldenkrais.com
Will send out a free packet of information on Feldenkrais and a list of practitioners in your area.

Homeopathy

American Institute of Homeopathy
1585 Glencoe St., Ste. 44
Denver, CO 80220-1338
(303) 321-4105

National Center for Homeopathy
801 North Fairfax St., Ste. 306
Alexandria, VA 22314
(703) 548-7790
Nonprofit educational organization that provides homeopathy information and training. It offers a $7.00
informational packet that includes a national directory of
practitioners, study groups, pharmacies, and resources. It
also sponsors an annual conference.

Massage

International Massage Association
P.O. Box 1400
Westminster, CO 80030-1400
1-800-776-6268
Referral service with names of massage therapists in
your area.
E-mail: massage@his.com
Server: internationalmassage.com

Osteopathy

American Osteopathic Association
142 East Ohio St.
Chicago, IL 60611
(312) 280-5800
Internet address: http://www.am-osteo-assn.org
Will give names of an affiliated osteopathic group in your area
and send out brochures about osteopathic medicine.

The American Academy of Osteopathy
3500 DePauw Blvd., Ste. 1080
Indianapolis, IN 46268-1139
(317) 879-1881
Will provide information on osteopaths who are board-
certified.

Rolfing

The Rolf Institute
205 Canyon Blvd.
Boulder, CO 80302-4920
(303) 449-5903
1-800-530-8875
Provides information on Rolfing and names of practitioners
in your area.

Website

Alternative medicine
http://www.halcyon.com/libastyr/netbib.html

✄
BENEFITS

Compensation Alert
843 2nd St.
Santa Rosa, CA 95404
(707) 545-2266
Nonprofit organization that provides assistance to workers, primarily in California, on worker's compensation and related issues. Publishes newsletter.

Consumer's Guide to Disability Insurance
Health Insurance Association of America
P.O. Box 41455
Washington, DC 20018
Write for free guide to disability insurance.

Medicare/Medicaid Programs
Health Care Financing Administration
Department of Health and Human Services
200 Independence Ave. SW
Washington, DC 20201
(202) 245-6113

National Association of Insurance Commissioners
120 West 12th St.
Kansas City, MO 64105
(816) 842-3600
Can provide you with number for your state insurance department.

National Insurance Consumers Organization
121 North Payne St.
Alexandria, VA 22314
(703) 549-8050
Provides referrals and advice to people with insurance complaints.

Social Security Administration
Office of Disability
Department of Health and Human Services
Altimeyer Building
6401 Security Blvd. #545
Baltimore, MD 21235
1-800-772-1213
(410) 965-3424
Internet address: http://www.ssa.gov/odhome/
Agency to contact if you want to apply for Social Security Disability. Call to request appropriate application forms. It provides a number of publications, including the *Social Security Handbook*, which summarizes information about federal disability, and a newsletter called "Disability Notes," which has articles on current disability issues.

✄

ERGONOMICS

Fax Response Ergonomic Database (FRED)
Ergodyne
140 Energy Park Dr., Ste. 1
St. Paul, MN 55108
1-800-373-3121
Outside United States and Canada: (612) 230-3813
Free service offering information on RSI, ergonomics, injury statistics, and regulatory information.
For hard copy, call 1-800-225-8238.

The Human Factors and Ergonomics Society
P.O. Box 1369
Santa Monica, California 90406-1369
(310) 394-1811

Fax: (310) 394-2410
Publishes newsletters and ergonomic information and has a
national listing of ergonomics professionals.

The National Institute for Occupational Safety and Health
4676 Columbia Parkway
Cincinnati, OH 45226
1-800-356-4674
NIOSH has released a 133-page primer outlining the
approaches used for identifying and correcting ergonomic
problems that is available free to the public.

✄
JOB ACCOMMODATION

American Occupational Therapy Association
1383 Picard Dr.
P.O. Box 1725
Rockville, MD 20849-1725
(301) 652-2682
(301) 652-7590
Refers employers and individuals to occupational therapists
who can help perform job analyses and design job accommodations.

Clearinghouse on Disability Information
Department of Education, OSERS
Switzer Building, #3132
Washington, DC 20202
1-800-458-5231

Job Accommodation Network
809 Allen Hall
West Virginia University
P.O. Box 6123
Morgantown, WV 26506-6123
1-800-526-7234
In Canada: 1-800-526-2262
In West Virginia: 1-800-526-4698
Information and consulting service providing individualized
job accommodations in response to inquiries.

**Northeast Disability and Business Technical
Assistance Center**
1-800-949-4232
Provides free information and training on the Americans
With Disabilities Act.

Rehabilitation International
25 E. 21st St.
New York, NY 10010
(212) 420-1500
Nonprofit organization that provides information on rehabilitation and prevention of disability.

✄

LEGAL RIGHTS AND ADA

American Bar Association
Commission on Mental and Physical Disability Law
1800 M St. NW
Washington, DC 20036
(202) 331-2240
Provides information and technical assistance on disability
law, as well as training on the ADA.

Department of Justice
Office on the Americans With Disabilities Act
P.O. Box 66118
Washington, DC 20035
(202) 514-2000

Disability Rights Education and Defense Fund Inc.
2212 Sixth St.
Berkeley, CA 94710
(510) 644-2555
Provides information on the Americans With Disabilities Act.

National Association of Social Security Claimants
1-800-431-2804

U.S. Equal Employment Opportunity Commission
Office of Communications and Legislative Affairs
1801 L St. NW
Washington, DC 20507
1-800-669-EEOC
Provides information on laws, including the Americans With Disabilities Act, enforced by the Equal Employment Opportunity Commission.

❡

MEDICAL ISSUES

Finding a Doctor

American Board of Medical Specialties
1-800-776-CERT
Lists board-certified doctors.

Requesting Records

Medical Information Bureau
P.O. Box 105 Essex Station
Boston, MA 02112
(617) 426-3660
The MIB discloses an individual's records for a fee of $8.00.

Treatment

National Organization of Neurological Disorders and Stroke
Bethesda, MD 20892
1-800-352-9424
Provides information on carpal tunnel syndrome and
chronic pain.

The Rehabilitation Accreditation Commission
4891 East Grant Rd.
Tucson, AZ 85712
(520) 325-1044
Provides a listing of pain-management programs.

U.S. Agency for Health Care Policy and Research Clearinghouse
P.O. Box 8546, Dept. P
Silver Spring, MD 20907
Offers a free booklet on questions to ask your doctor before
surgery, as well as on pain control after surgery.

NEWSLETTERS AND MAILING LISTS

Association for Disability Rights in the Workplace Inc.
3720 Jay Lane
Spring Hill, TN 37174
(615) 486-1688
Nonprofit organization that publishes a newsletter on disabled workers' rights.

CTD News
747 Dresher Rd.
P.O. Box 980
Horsham, PA 19044-0980
(215) 784-0860
E-mail: mgauf@lrp.com.
Monthly newsletter published by LRP Publications and the Center for Workplace Health Information. Well-written and up to date, it contains a variety of news on RSI developments.

Ergonomics News
1100 Superior Ave.
Cleveland, OH 4414-2543

Healthy Office Report
Courthouse Place
54 W. Hubbard St., Ste. 403
Chicago, IL 60610
Monthly newsletter aimed at clerical professions. Includes coverage of RSI.

Mouth: The Voice of Disability Rights
61 Brighton St.
Rochester, NY 14607
(716) 473-6764

RSI East
This is an East Coast mailing list for people with RSI. Send
e-mail to listserv@juvm.stjohns.edu with message reading
"subscribe rsi-east" and your name.

The RSI Network
970 Paradise Way
Palo Alto, CA 94306
Contact: Caroline Rose
Available on CompuServe. Type "gozmc:downtech" and look
for "rsinet.sea."
To subscribe, send a mail message to
majordomo@world.std.com. Put "subscribe rsi" on the
message line.

Sorehand
This is a San Francisco-based listserv mailing list for people
with RSI. To subscribe, send E-mail to listserv@vm.ucsf.edu.
Message should read "subscribe sorehand" with your name.

Workers Health International Newsletter
P.O. Box 199
Sheffield, SI IFQ England
0114-276-5695

❧
POLITICAL ADVOCACY

Massachusetts Coalition on New Office Technology (CNOT)
650 Beacon St., 5th Floor
Boston, MA 02215
(617) 247-6827
This group has a hotline with medical and legal referrals and
technical information on RSI. It also has a library, provides

ergonomic training, and staffs RSI ACTION, a project that runs RSI support groups and advocacy efforts for injured and at-risk office workers.

Also see COSH groups under *Workplace Safety*.

❊
PSYCHOTHERAPY

American Psychiatric Association
(202) 682-6000

American Psychological Association
(202) 336-5700

National Association of Social Workers
(202) 408-8600

National Mental Health Association (NMHA)
1021 Price St.
Alexandria, VA 22314
1-800-228-1114
Provides information on how to find treatment in your area.

❊
SUPPORT GROUPS

American Self-Help Clearinghouse
St. Clares-Riverside Medical Center
25 Pocono Rd.
Denville, NJ 07834
(201) 625-7101
(201) 625-9565
Provides information on finding or forming a support group.

Association for Repetitive Motion Syndromes (A.R.M.S.)
P.O. Box 514
Santa Rosa, CA 95402
(707) 571-0397
Provides information, research updates, seminars, and information on support groups. The newsletter is particularly helpful, with names and numbers of support groups throughout the country, as well as useful tips for people with RSI.

National Coalition of Injured Workers
12 Rejane St.
Coventry, RI 02816
(401) 828-6520
Provides referrals to a contact group in your area that can help give you advice on the worker's compensation system and support groups.

Women's RSI Support Team Inc.
263 Brunswick St., 2nd Floor
Fitzroy 3065
Australia

✂ VOCATIONAL REHABILITATION

National Rehabilitation Information Center (NARIC)
8455 Colesville Rd., Ste. 935
Silver Spring, MD 20910-3319
1-800-346-2742
(301) 588-9284
Website: http://www.naric.com/naric
Has more than 50,000 documents on disability and rehabilitation.

Student Support Services Project Grants
U.S. Department of Education
Postsecondary Education
400 Maryland Ave. SW
Washington, DC 20202-5446
(202) 708-4804
Provides assistance to disabled students.

U.S. Department of Education
Postsecondary Education
400 Maryland Ave. SW
Washington, DC 20202-5446
(202) 708-4690
Government agency that offers educational opportunity
grants to provide assistance to eligible undergraduate students
with financial need.

�֎ WORKPLACE SAFETY

AFL-CIO
815 16th St. NW
Washington, DC 20006
(202) 637-5376
The AFL-CIO has launched a "Stop the Pain" campaign that
focuses on RSIs in the workplace. It has a variety of information available, including a report on RSI and a "Workplace
Ergo Action Kit."

Campaign for VDT Safety
9 to 5 National Association of Working Women
614 Superior Ave. NW
Cleveland, OH 44113
(216) 566-9308
Hotline: 1-800-245-9825
9 to 5 has done extensive research on a variety of workplace issues, including RSI, and has published reports that are available to the public. It also operates a job problem hotline.

Canadian Centre for Occupational Health and Safety
250 Main St. East
Hamilton, Ontario L8N 1H6
In Canada: 1-800-263-8466
(416) 572-4500

Communication Workers of America
501 Third St. NW
Washington, DC 20003
(202) 434-1160
CWA has been one of the main groups on the forefront of research into RSI and VDT safety. It works with other unions on training, education, and lobbying and provides resource information to the public.

Labor Occupational Health Program
Center for Occupational and Environmental Health
University of California Berkeley
(510) 642-5507
Offers health and safety training, as well as information and technical assistance to workers and health professionals.

National Institute of Occupational Safety and Health
4676 Columbia Parkway
Cincinnati, OH 45226
1-800-35-NIOSH
Federally funded U.S. government research group that provides free information, as well as free literature searches on RSI.

National Safe Workplace Institute
122 South Michigan Ave., Ste. 1450
Chicago, IL 60603
(312) 939-0690

Occupational Safety and Health Administration
Website: http://www.osha.gov
Website has listings of programs in various regions.

Worksafe!
c/o San Francisco Labor Council
510 Harrison St.
San Francisco, CA 94105
(415) 433-5977

�֍

COSH GROUPS

Alaska

Alaska Health Project
218 East 4th Ave.
Anchorage, AK 99501
(907) 276-2864

California

Los Angeles COSH (LACOSH)
5855 Venice Blvd.
Los Angeles, CA 90016
(213) 931-9000

Sacramento COSH (SACOSH)
c/o Fire Fighters, Local 522
3101 Stockton Blvd.
Sacramento, CA 95820
(916) 442-4390

Santa Clara COSH (SCCOSH)
760 N. First St.
San Jose, CA 95112
(408) 998-4050

Worksafe/Francis Schreiberg
c/o San Francisco Labor Council
660 Howard St., 3rd Floor
San Francisco, CA 94105
(415) 543-2699

Connecticut

Connecticut COSH (CONNCOSH)
77 Huyshoup Ave., 2nd Floor
Hartford, CT 06106
(860) 549-1877

District of Columbia

Alice Hamilton Occupational Health Center
410 Seventh St. SE
Washington, DC 20003
(202) 543-0005/(301) 731-8530

Illinois

Chicago Area COSH (CACOSH)
847 W. Jackson Blvd., 7th Floor
Chicago, IL 60607
(312) 996-3228

Maine

Maine Labor Group on Health
Box V
Augusta, ME 04330
(207) 622-7823

Massachusetts

**Massachusetts Coalition for Occupational Safety and Health
(MASSCOSH)**
555 Amory St.
Boston, MA 02130
(617) 524-6686
E-mail: 71112.600@compuserve.com
Western MASSCOSH
458 Bridge St.
Springfield, MA
(413) 247-9413
E-mail: masscosh@external.umass.edu

Michigan

Southeast Michigan COSH (SEMCOSH)
1550 Howard St.
Detroit, MI 48216
(313) 961-3345

Minnesota

MNCOSH
c/o Lyle Krych
5013 Girard Ave. N
Minneapolis, MN 55430
(612) 572-6997

New Hampshire

NHCOSH
110 Sheep Davis Rd.
Pembroke, NH 03275
(603) 226-0516

New York

Alleghany (ALCOSH)
100 East Second St.
Jamestown, NY 14701
(716) 488-0720

Central New York (CNYCOSH)
615 W. Genessee St.
Syracuse, NY 13204
(315) 471-6187
E-mail: eameltz@mailboxsyr.edu

Eastern New York (ENYCOSH)
c/o Larry Rafferty
121 Erie Blvd.
Schenectady, NY 12305
(518) 372-4308

New York (NYCOSH)
275 Seventh Ave., 8th Floor
New York, NY 10001
(212) 627-3900
(914) 939-5612 (Lower Hudson)
(516) 273-1234 (Long Island)
E-mail: 71112.1020@compuserve.com

Rochester (ROCOSH)
46 Prince St.
Rochester, NY 14607
(716) 244-0420
E-mail: SPULA@DBI.cc.Rochester.edu

Western New York (WNYCOSH)
2495 Main St., Ste. 438
Buffalo, NY 14214
(716) 833-5416

North Carolina

North Carolina COSH
P.O. Box 2514
Durham, NC 27705
(919) 286-9249
E-mail: HN2100@Handsnet.org

Oregon

ICWU-Portland,
c/o Dick Edgington
7440 SW 87th St.
Portland, OR 07223
(503) 244-8429

Pennsylvania

Philadelphia COSH (PHILACOSH)
3001 Walnut St., 5th Floor
Philadelphia, PA 19104
(215) 386-7000

Rhode Island

Rhode Island COSH
741 Westminster St.
Providence, RI 02903
(401) 751-2015

Texas

TEXCOSH
c/o Karyl Dunson
5735 Regina
Beaumont, TX 77706
(409) 898-1427

Washington

WASHCOSH
6770 E. Marginal Way S.
Seattle, WA 98108
(206) 767-7426

Wisconsin

Wisconsin COSH (WISCOSH)
734 N. 26th St.
Milwaukee, WI 53230
(414) 933-2338

OTHER GROUPS

Arthritis Foundation
1314 Spring St. NW
Atlanta, GA 30309
1-800-283-7800
A nonprofit organization, with chapters throughout the United States, which funds research and provides programs and services for people affected by rheumatic disease. Some chapters also provide information and support groups on RSI. One of those is the Long Island Arthritis Foundation; (516) 427-8272.

American Chronic Pain Association
P.O. Box 850
Rocklin, CA 95677
(916) 632-0922
A nonprofit organization that provides information, seminars, and support groups for people with chronic pain.

London Hazards Centre
Interchange Studios
Dalby St.
London, NWS 3NQ, England
0171-267-3387
E-mail: lonhaz@mcri.poptel.org.uk

Workers Institute for Occupational Safety and Health
1126 16th St., NW, Room 403
Washington, DC 20036
(202) 887-0191

Worksafe Australia
National Occupational Health and Safety Commission
92 Parramatta Rd.
Camperdown NSW 2001
Austrailia
(02) 565-9555

GLOSSARY

Abduction Moving away from the median plane of the body.

Acupressure A Chinese healing art similar to acupuncture, except that fingertip pressure rather than needles is used to relieve symptoms. It can be useful in relieving trigger points, which are knotted muscles that can be painful when touched.

Acupuncture An ancient Chinese healing art that seeks to remove energy blockages in the body by applying gentle pressure with tiny, sterilized needles. It is used to relieve symptoms, as well as promote general well-being. Research has shown that acupuncture releases endorphins, the body's natural painkillers.

Acute pain Severe pain following a trauma that generally lasts for a relatively short period of time.

Alexander Technique A system of retraining the body to avoid unhealthy postures. Its underlying theory is that the body assumes unnatural and unhealthy postures in response to stresses.

Americans With Disabilities Act Federal law prohibiting discrimination against disabled workers in hiring or in the workplace.

Biofeedback Relaxation therapy in which you are hooked up, usually by electrodes, to a machine that monitors heart rate, body temperature, and muscle tension. Through visual or auditory cues, it helps you control your physiological responses to stress.

Bursitis   Inflammation of the bursa, which is a fluid-filled sac that acts as a cushion in the shoulder joint. Symptoms include pain and swelling. It is associated with frequent overhead reaching and is generally not considered a serious condition.

Carpal tunnel syndrome   The most well-known form of Repetitive Strain Injury, it is the constellation of symptoms occurring as a result of the compression of the median nerve, which runs through the wrist to the fingers. When it is work-related, it is associated with excessive up-and-down motions of the wrist.

Chronic pain   Pain that continues or recurs over a long period.

Contrast bath   Therapeutic method in which the hands and arms are immersed first in warm water and then in cold water at intervals to reduce pain and promote circulation.

Cortisone   Hormone produced by the cortex of the adrenal gland that can be produced synthetically. It is used for its anti-inflammatory effect.

De Quervain's disease   Named for Swiss surgeon Fritz De Quervain, it's a form of tendinitis at the base of the thumb.

Disability insurance   Insurance that can be purchased privately or through a job to reimburse a worker for wages lost as a result of being unable to continue working.

Dorsal   Pertaining to the back, or posterior. When used in reference to the hand, it refers to the back of the hand.

Electromyograph   A machine commonly referred to as an EMG that uses electrical stimulation of the nerves to test neuromuscular activity.

Endorphins   Natural painkillers produced by the human nervous system.

Ergonomics   Science of adapting tools and equipment to the human body. A multidisciplinary specialty, it involves knowledge of human anatomy, biomechanics, psychology, and industrial engineering.

Extension   Bending up.

Feldenkrais   A system of body work and gentle exercise aimed at achieving better posture and coordination. Its primary goal is to teach greater body awareness.

Flexion   Bending down.

Flotation therapy   Relaxation therapy using a tank filled with highly salted water so that the body floats. It provides an environment of restricted light and sound and is used to treat people with chronic pain, among other things.

Ganglion cyst   Swelling under the skin, usually at a joint capsule or tendon sheath. It can disappear or recur of its own accord and is considered benign. It may be painful.

Homeopathy   Based on the notion that physical symptoms are part of the body's own defense system, this therapy uses substances called tinctures, highly diluted and shaken extracts of natural ingredients to treat illness.

Hyperextension   Position of maximum bending up at a joint.

Imprinting   Theory of pain in which it is believed that pain is stamped onto the nervous system, which retains a memory of the pain even after the injurious activity has ceased.

Inflammation   Reaction of tissues to infection or trauma, characterized by warmth, swelling, redness, and pain.

Lordosis   Natural curvature of the neck/lumbar spine, shaped like a sea horse.

Lyme disease   An acute, recurring inflammatory infection that is contracted via a tick bite. Its symptoms mimic those of some RSIs.

Myotherapy   Series of firm, manual techniques in which sustained pressure is applied to trigger points to relieve pain and spasm.

Neurologist   Medical doctor who specializes in problems of the nervous system.

NSAIDs   Nonsteroidal anti-inflammatory drugs, prescribed for pain.

Occupational therapist   Medical specialist who helps reduce pain and focuses on helping a patient accomplish tasks of day-to-day living by providing adaptive aids or devising other ways to accomplish the tasks.

Orthopedist Surgically oriented medical doctor who is a specialist in muscles, joints, and bones.

Osteopathy A therapeutic approach that uses the usual forms of medical therapy, but which emphasizes the relationship of the musculoskeletal system and the organs. Osteopaths use a range of manipulative techniques to relieve pain and restore mobility.

Palpate To use the fingers or hands to examine.

Paraffin bath Heated metal container filled with melted paraffin, or wax, and wintergreen oil that is used to get deep heat to the muscles and tendons of the hands.

Physiatrist Medical doctor who specializes in physical medicine and rehabilitation.

Physical therapist Medical specialist who focuses on reducing pain, restoring strength, and preventing further loss of function.

Pronation Turning the palm down.

Psychogenic Of mental or emotional origin.

Psychotherapist A professional who counsels patients on mental-health problems. Psychotherapists include psychiatrists, psychologists, clinical social workers, psychiatric nurses, and individuals trained in counseling.

Radial tunnel syndrome Entrapment of the radial nerve caused by twisting your arm frequently and forcefully.

Raynaud's disease Constriction of the blood vessels that causes the fingers to become cold and pale and eventually, loss of sensation in the hands.

Referred pain Phenomenon in which injury is in one part of the body, but pain is felt elsewhere.

Rheumatologist Medical doctor who is a specialist in the inflammation or degeneration of connective tissue and related structures in the body.

Rolfing   Technique of deep body massage intended to help realign the body by changing the length and tone of muscle tissue.

Static muscle loading   Maintaining the muscles in a prolonged state of isometric contraction. As a result, blood circulation is decreased and waste products are not removed from the blood, leading to muscle soreness.

Subluxation   A term frequently used by chiropractors to describe defective joint movement.

Supination   Turning the palm up.

Tendinitis   Inflammation of a tendon that includes microtears in the fibers of the tendon.

Tendon   Ropelike band that connects muscle to bone. Acting like a pulley, it transfers force from muscle to bone during movement.

Tenosynovitis   Inflammation of the fluid-filled sheath, called the synovium, which surrounds the tendon.

TENS   Transcutaneous electrical nerve stimulator, or TENS, used to relieve pain by transmitting a low-level electrical impulse from a small box through wires to electrodes taped to the injured area.

Therapeutic touch   A system of balancing the energy fields of the human body without actually touching it.

Thoracic outlet syndrome   Compression of the nerves and blood vessels between the neck and shoulder. It has been associated with unbalanced posture, related to a tight pectoralis minor muscle. It also has been linked to certain chronic diseases and congenital defects, such as an extra rib.

Tricyclic antidepressant   Drug that is used to treat depression. It also alleviates pain.

Trigger finger   A form of tenosynovitis in which the inflamed synovium is so swollen that it restricts movement of the tendon in your finger, making it difficult to straighten the finger after it is bent.

Trigger point   A point of knotted muscles that is particularly sensitive to touch, and may be experienced as stabbing pain when touched.

Ulnar deviation   Bending the wrist toward the finger.

Ultrasound   Sound waves at the very high frequency of more than 20,000 vibrations per second. It is used in a machine that is applied to injured areas that have been lubricated with a gel to provide deep heat and stimulation to muscles and tendons.

VDT   Video display terminal.

Visualization   A technique used in hypnosis in which subject imagines being in a pleasant, restful place. It is used to promote relaxation and reduce pain.

Worker's compensation   System of no-fault insurance regulated by the government that reimburses workers for injuries or illnesses incurred on the job.

Writer's cramp   Involuntary cramping of the hand and forearm. Also known as focal dystonia. It can occur after prolonged handwriting with an overly thin pencil or pen.

INDEX

✄